A Beginner's Guide to Cognitive Analytic Therapy

This text provides an accessible, reader-friendly guide to conducting Cognitive Analytic Therapy (CAT) on a one-to-one basis, developed in partnership with service users who have lived experience of CAT.

The book will cover the applications of CAT in clinical practice including: assessment; introducing CAT; the main concepts and how to build a therapeutic relationship; mapping; the middle phase and the integration of other models; monitoring; developing exits; the ending and saying goodbye. Grounded in CAT theory, the content will be ordered sequentially, as one would conduct the therapy, and will feature first-hand accounts from CAT-experienced service users including their own perspectives on the model and the impact it had on their wellbeing.

A straightforward, beginner's introduction to practicing CAT, this book will be useful for trainee practitioners, assistant and trainee clinical/counselling psychologists, and those practising CAT-informed therapy in supervision.

Sarah Craven-Staines is a Clinical Psychologist and CAT Practitioner with more than 20 years of experience working within the field of mental health. She is a Senior Fellow of the Higher Education Academy, working for the Doctorate in Clinical Psychology course at Teesside University and offering CAT in a clinical setting.

Jayne Finch is a Clinical Psychologist and CAT Practitioner, having worked in the NHS for 20 years, predominantly within Adult Mental Health Services. She now works in a Clinical Tutor role for the Doctorate in Clinical Psychology course at Teesside University, as well as conducting CAT clinically.

'This excellent volume offers an invaluable and overdue addition to the CAT literature. Its clear focus and description of the key features of the model as used in "front line" clinical work along with its focus on "lived experience" of the approach from both practitioners and, importantly, service users is engaging and inspiring. The prominent voice of "service users", who give personal accounts of therapy in the context of their overall journey, is illuminating, brave, and moving and is an especially helpful and relevant feature of the book. They also exemplify and illustrate the "genuinely collaborative" nature of the CAT approach. The book will undoubtedly be of considerable usefulness not only to CAT trainees and practitioners but to many others, including potentially those who might engage with CAT (clients, patients, service users), and potentially beyond to anyone concerned with mental health problems and their treatment. This should include senior health service managers, service commissioners and funding agencies, media, and also those active in the broader public and socio-political domain.'

Ian B. Kerr, MD, *Consultant Psychiatrist and Medical Psychotherapist, Te Whatu Ora-Health NZ, Whangārei, Honorary Senior Lecturer, Department of Psychological Medicine, Waipapa Taumata Rau-University of Auckland*

'This a thorough and well-arranged, distinctive introduction to the ideas and methods of Cognitive Analytic Therapy. It gives a rich and lucid account of all the steps to and aspects of the traditional CAT approach to a time-limited, brief focused psychotherapy. It locates CAT as a cognitive therapy and should work well as a guide to beginners in therapy, especially those meeting CAT for the first time as part of their clinical psychology training. It is distinctive and innovative in building the book around the perspectives and experiences of two clients of psychotherapy. Anyone who wants to join the conversation about how to understand and apply CAT should find this book a good beginning.'

Steve Potter, *Psychotherapist who teaches and supervises Cognitive Analytic Therapy (CAT) and its application to reflective practice in the UK and internationally*

'The authors of this book set out to produce a user friendly clinician's "how to do it" guide to Cognitive Analytic Therapy and they have achieved their aim. They cover all the basics but also mention new developments that therapists could experiment with as they become more confident. The inclusion of two service users as fellow authors is a valuable addition to previous books where we only get brief snapshots of service user experiences. Really helpful to follow the service user experience through from start to finish.'

Dr Alison Jenaway, *previously Consultant Psychiatrist in Medical Psychotherapy (now retired), CAT Therapist and Supervisor, past Chair of ACAT*

'With recent rises in mental health problems, there is a growing need to train more therapists. For those coming to CAT for the first time, their first experiences of the model have the power to spark curiosity and a thirst to learn more. This book has much to offer as the first step into Cognitive Analytic Therapy. It bridges the gap of offering an accessible first step into the CAT literature combined with hearing real and grounded experiences of having CAT. At its heart CAT is a collaborative model and it is this joint endeavour, giving voice to those who have generously shared their stories which makes this book truly special.'

Dr Jenny Marshall, *Consultant Psychologist and Joint Trustwide Lead for CAT*

A Beginner's Guide to Cognitive Analytic Therapy

Practitioner and Service User Perspectives

Sarah Craven-Staines and Jayne Finch

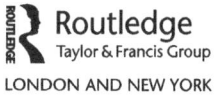

Routledge
Taylor & Francis Group

LONDON AND NEW YORK

Designed cover image: Andrew Forcer

First published 2024
by Routledge
4 Park Square, Milton Park, Abingdon, Oxon OX14 4RN

and by Routledge
605 Third Avenue, New York, NY 10158

Routledge is an imprint of the Taylor & Francis Group, an informa business

British Library Cataloguing-in-Publication Data
A catalogue record for this book is available from the British Library

Library of Congress Cataloging-in-Publication Data
Names: Craven-Staines, Sarah, author. | Finch, Jayne, author.
Title: A beginner's guide to cognitive analytic therapy : practitioner and service user perspectives / Sarah Craven-Staines, Jayne Finch.
Description: Abingdon, Oxon ; New York, NY : Routledge, 2024. |
Includes bibliographical references and index. |
Identifiers: LCCN 2023059292 (print) | LCCN 2023059293 (ebook) |
ISBN 9781032311425 (hardback) | ISBN 9781032311333 (paperback) |
ISBN 9781003308256 (ebook) Subjects: LCSH: Cognitive-analytic therapy. |
Psychotherapists--Training of. | Psychotherapy--Methodology.
Classification: LCC RC489.C6 C73 2024 (print) | LCC RC489.C6 (ebook) |
DDC 616.89/14--dc23/eng/20240123
LC record available at https://lccn.loc.gov/2023059292
LC ebook record available at https://lccn.loc.gov/2023059293

ISBN: 978-1-032-31142-5 (hbk)
ISBN: 978-1-032-31133-3 (pbk)
ISBN: 978-1-003-30825-6 (ebk)

DOI: 10.4324/9781003308256

Typeset in Times New Roman
by SPi Technologies India Pvt Ltd (Straive)

Contents

Acknowledgements

First and foremost, we would like to acknowledge all of the service users we have worked with throughout our careers; we have been honoured to share in your stories and journeys in the work we have done together. Learning is a reciprocal process, and we have learnt as much from you as we hope you have learnt from CAT.

We would like to take this opportunity to wholeheartedly thank Karen and Andrew, who have been involved in the process of writing this book. We have greatly valued your ability to share as openly and emotively as you have done, and we feel hugely privileged to have you involved all the way through the process. Andrew, you have done a fantastic job in designing the front cover of this book. What a talent you have; we are so grateful! We also want to acknowledge the therapists who have both provided consent to share their CAT tools developed in therapy with Karen and Andrew. You know who you are, and we thank you!

We have both worked for a number of years within the North East and feel that we have been supervised and taught CAT by one of the best, Dr Kate Freshwater. We thank you for your continued encouragement and belief in us over the years! We also want to thank our wonderful colleague and friend Dr Lisa Caygill; you have kept us going all the way through with your positive comments, and your proofreading has been incredible!

The process of writing this book has been long and time consuming, and one which we couldn't do without the consistent love, encouragement and backing of our close friends and family. Our girls have enjoyed many a 'book writing' day spent playing together! Girls, this is for you, and we love you always. Our husbands have been amazing, keeping the family ships afloat as we have been on our voyage of writing. We are so thankful for you both. Last, but by no means least, a huge thank you to our parents for being there all throughout our lives, supporting us through training, more training, even more training, and our career paths; that takes great commitment, so thank you always!

Foreword

This is an excellent read for all students training in CAT. It is written by two experienced professionals who are both therapists and trainers, who know their subject well and clearly rejoice in CAT's flexibility. The book is particularly strong on emphasising the wide range of choices of therapeutic approaches within the CAT framework. It encourages practitioners to bring their own individual strengths into their work. This helps what can often be a daunting task of learning a new approach to therapy, particularly one with many different written structures such as CAT. It offers a flexibility to work with what both therapist and patient can manage in the here and now. Sometimes a patient may make only one small change, but it might be a small change that is, for them, heroic. The careful description of the different stages of working from the CAT model are well described and easy to read. They also include a really helpful chapter on the potential challenges of working with the CAT model and offer suggestions for understanding and resolve.

One of the great strengths of the book is the contribution of two service users about their own experiences of CAT and the effect on their symptoms and lives in general. These accounts are threaded through all sections which make the text grounded and real. They contain details of their journeys, their difficulties and breakthroughs.

Karen writes ten years on from her CAT therapy: 'Even today I remind myself that I don't need to be perfect, and I still hear my therapists voice reminding me of "Good Enough"'.

Andrew writes: 'I had a full course of CAT which I feel gave me the tools to finally get to grips with my issues. CAT gave me a road map, or as I refer to it, an internal sat-nav. I don't remember a lot of the details of each session, but I do recall them being hard work.' Later he writes: 'I can say now that this therapy saved my life.'

This is a well prepared and thoughtful contribution to the literature on CAT and will be of great value to students.

Elizabeth Wilde McCormick, MA psych. Dip.soc.psych.

Founder member and Life Member of the Association for Cognitive Analytic Therapy. Author of *Change for the Better: Personal development through practical psychotherapy* now in its 5th edition.

Book review

This book concerns the delivery of cognitive analytic therapy for those that are interested in training in this model of psychotherapy or have started their training. Cognitive analytic therapy (CAT) is an avowedly integrative therapy and therefore therapists need to finely balance and incorporate both cognitive and analytic concepts and practices into their work whilst helping people. This book has nicely sensed the challenge of that and equally concerns itself with both analytic and cognitive aspects without neglecting or infantilising the other. The 'tools' of CAT are fully explained as well as how to use them well sensitively and in a person-centred manner.

CAT is quite a technical psychotherapy and for the model to be done competently, then trainees and newcomers need to be on top of the technical aspects in order that the relational aspects can come to life in the consulting room. This book is good at demystifying the language and technical aspects of CAT and therefore will support the learning of trainees and newcomers. Each chapter has a useful practical tone to it that will support the transfer of theoretical concepts into practice and will help trainees and newcomers internalise the methods and the therapy. The book retains its user-friendliness throughout.

The authors have clearly spent a lot of time talking with two ex-CAT patients and with many ex and current trainees to produce the book and you can hear their voices and influences throughout the sixteen chapters. The three-phase (reformulation, recognition and revision) approach to CAT is well represented and balanced across these chapters.

This is a practical and not an academic textbook and it is all the better for that, as it couches itself in a relational model and attempts to bring to life the complex relational aspects of CAT work in an accessible and easy to apply manner.

Dr Stephen Kellett, CAT psychotherapist, CBT psychotherapist, Consultant Clinical Psychologist and Research Director; Rotherham Doncaster and South Humber NHS Foundation Trust.

Preface

Both Sarah and Jayne were introduced to Cognitive Analytic Therapy (CAT) during their Doctorate in Clinical Psychology training at Teesside University, between 2004 and 2007. They both found the accessibility of the model and its collaborative, relational approach in practice important in their foundations as developing practitioners. Over the course of their years in practice (and subsequent training as CAT practitioners), they have frequently been aware of the difficulty in comprehending the CAT literature for those new to the approach. Through supervising trainee clinical psychologists, using a CAT informed approach, Sarah and Jayne have often found themselves wishing for a more user-friendly, simple-to-use, academic text, to help explain some of the complex concepts of CAT. As they both now work in academia alongside their clinical work, they took the opportunity to blend both aspects of their working lives and to write this book, which they have felt has long been needed in the discipline of CAT. They hope it will be of much use to those new to CAT, training in the approach, or supervising therapists practicing the model.

1 The introduction

Where we began

As we start to put pen to paper, we felt it pertinent to share a little of ourselves, our own experiences and what led us to the point of wanting to write a book for those of you interested in beginning to use Cognitive Analytic Therapy (CAT). Our first 'writing' meeting took place in a little café called The Scene, an irony not lost on us as we began to think about how best to set the scene to this beginner's guide for you, the reader. We began by reflecting upon our own journeys into practising CAT. Interestingly, we found that our first acquaintances with CAT were quite similar, having both observed experienced CAT practitioners utilise the model in practice. Whether this was the clarity that emerged when watching a supervisor tentatively map out patterns, the insight that was gained when considering a cognitive behavioural therapy case from a different position or the experience of having a specialist CAT placement during clinical psychology training. From observing the use of CAT 'live', we were quickly 'hooked' as we could see its potential benefit and applicability for those we worked with.

Similarly, for both of us, our reading around CAT came later. We often found that the literature underpinning the model was dense to start with, and until our knowledge of the model grew, it was difficult to understand the jargon that came with CAT, or how other models were integrated within its development. We were drawn to articles such as Chess Denman's (2001) paper, in which CAT was made more accessible and tangible for those starting out. It was this literature that left us wondering: would it be possible to write a book which made the areas that we initially found tricky in CAT, easier to understand?

It was in part this struggle that led us to where we are today; starting to write this book in the hope that it allows those beginning their CAT journey to feel able to grasp an early understanding, before making their way into the wealth of literature that awaits them. Our passion and drive to advocate for CAT in practice has continued throughout our years of using the model. We hope that this text reflects our enthusiasm but does so in a way that is realistic and open, highlighting the strengths of the approach as well as the areas of continuing development, challenge and adaptation. Our ultimate aspiration is to do

DOI: 10.4324/9781003308256-1

justice to Ryle's early vision of CAT as an easily accessible model for the multidisciplinary staff who access and practice it.

A core premise of CAT is that it should occupy a space that is truly collaborative and relational, aspiring to hold the therapeutic relationship in mind at all times and sitting side by side with the service user in working together to understand their difficulties and take steps forward. We hope that this book is also experienced relationally, as we aim to sit side by side with you, the reader, in considering the key areas of CAT.

A truly relational book wouldn't be possible without the involvement of those who have experienced the therapeutic relationship from a service user perspective. We have collaborated with two people in the writing of this book, namely, Karen and Andrew, who have at various points in their lives been service users (a term they have chosen) and who have provided an open and honest account of their own experiences of CAT. They provide an invaluable insight into the parts of therapy that worked well for them, and the areas which they found more difficult. We recognise that people's personal experience of CAT will be varied, depending on their readiness for change, the individual experiences leading them to therapy, and how safe they felt within the therapy and the therapeutic relationship (to name just a few factors!). As such, we want to highlight that the service users' perspectives within this book are their own, subjective encounters, which they have taken great courage in sharing, and for which we are truly thankful. Naturally, whilst personal accounts cannot be generalised to all who experience CAT, we hope that their explanations do resonate with you as practising therapists and give food for thought in terms of areas which we need to be mindful of as clinicians. In addition, we hope that their involvement in the book will enable us to consider CAT from a critical perspective, promoting our thinking about areas in which the model can improve and be developed in the future.

Often, the terms 'service user' and 'therapist' come with the connotation of a 'them and us' attitude. We would like to explicitly challenge this position. We all live with varying degrees of physical and mental wellness; therefore, throughout life and due to our experiences, we may encounter times in which we suffer both physical and/or mental 'ill' health. We are all users of services within our own right. Therapists, just like everyone else, will at times be on the receiving end of physical or mental healthcare. Whilst training in CAT mandates the need for the trainee practitioner to have their own therapy, we would invite you not to see this as a 'tick box' exercise. As practitioners, we too have our own narratives and experiences – those that are healthy and those which might involve our suffering. We too are the service users, yet we have the privilege of being trained in a therapy to help understand the complexities of the mind. Our aim as the 'therapist', then, is to help the service user become *their own* therapist. Whilst as staff we may continue to encounter the 'them and us' attitude at times in the services we work within, we would encourage you to hold in mind that we are all human and to address and challenge this outlook whenever possible as we strive to work in therapy as equals.

Karen reflects here on her motivation for being involved in the book:

> *...it felt important to be a part of the book so that people can read it and see that real people have had it and how it benefitted them, because it's alright, the therapist saying this is what it is and this is what you get from it, but I think you need the true version of what the service user went through and the benefits it had to them to make them realise that actually it really, really, worked and I think it's also important that we highlight what an emotional roller coaster it can be as well.*

Andrew says:

> *It's good to be involved so people can see, and again I don't want to sound melodramatic, but there is light at the end of the tunnel, there is a way through this, and you can lead a pretty normal life because of it. And I think anything where service users are involved is a good thing, you know.*

The evidence base

As the intention of this book is to provide you with a 'how-to' of delivering CAT, we will not focus too heavily upon the theory and research which underpins the model. Yet a moment does need to be taken to acknowledge its importance and the need for ongoing exploration in the future. There is a growing body of articles which report the advancing evidence base and development of the model, which began initially in the early 1980s with Anthony Ryle. The Salkovskis (1995, in Feltham & Horton, 2012) hourglass model proposes a three-stage approach to developing the evidence base for new therapies, which includes case reports and single case designs, randomised controlled trials (RCTs), service evaluations and field experiments. It is well documented within the CAT literature that the model to date has a greater association with practice-based evidence than with evidence-based practice. Whilst some randomised controlled trials for CAT are now published, the ongoing popularity of CAT in routine practice means that greater support for its use and effectiveness has emerged through these means rather than through the use of RCTs (Ryle et al., 2014). Despite its relative lack of an evidence base, CAT has continued to hold its place in practice and is consistently popular amongst therapists due to its recognition and value within the workplace. Figure 1.1 provides a timeline of the development of CAT, beginning with the thinking that paved the way prior to its fundamental 'birth' in 1984, right up to the present day.

Originally, CAT was designed by Anthony Ryle as a solution to the problem of a busy GP practice, in which he began to make links between physical and

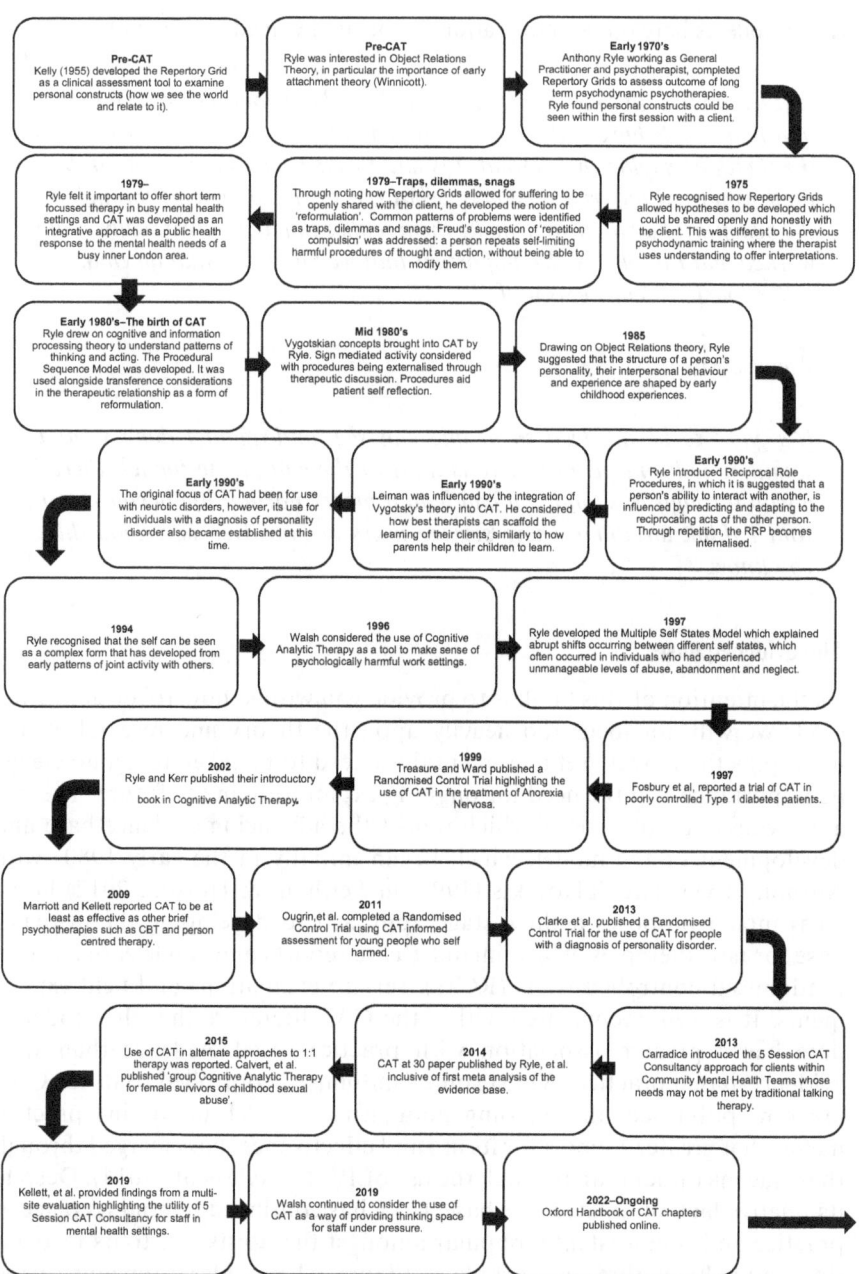

Figure 1.1 The history of CAT, before, then and now.

emotional health. The CAT model was intended to be a short-term approach to understanding emotional difficulties from an integrative perspective, utilising object relations theory, cognitive theory and personal construct theory, to name a few. The short-term approach to therapy evolved, within which structured one-to-one sessions included assessment, reformulation, intervention and evaluation phases.

Over the course of nearly 40 years of CAT in practice, its use has become more influential, not only on a one-to-one basis, but also for service users whose needs may not be best met by a traditional talking therapy (through five-session CAT consultancy, Carradice, 2013), and in support of mental health practitioners (through mapping team dynamics organisationally). Literature reports its use not only for varied diagnostic presentations, but also across the lifespan and for individuals with a learning disability. The utility of CAT is diverse, and its flexibility, creativity and variety mean that it can be adaptable to a wide range of needs. Developing skill as a CAT practitioner to adapt the model to meet the service user's requirements can be anxiety provoking and may take time, good supervision and experience; however, it does allow for a greater person-centred style of care, rather than expecting the service user to flex to fit within a manualised approach.

Power, difference and diversity

CAT is a collaborative therapy with the therapeutic relationship at its heart. In taking a "radically social" (Ryle & Kerr, 2002, p. 21) perspective on the development of the self, it could be argued that the approach strives to consider the socio-political context of the individual, to a greater degree than many other models of one-to-one talking therapy. In their introductory text, Ryle and Kerr (2002) recognise the effects of early deprivation and trauma on mental health, including the impact of being brought up in "low status, socio-economic groups". In more recent years, the evidence surrounding the impact of Adverse Childhood Experiences (ACEs, Felitti et al., 1998) on later health and wellbeing has reinforced this relationship. Models such as the Power Threat Meaning Framework (Johnstone et al., 2018) have gone some way in operationalising these understandings, making greater sense of the impact of various types of power on the individual. Ryle and Kerr (2002, p. 38) also argued that "some form of culture mapping should be at least implicit within any model of psychotherapy" and that "CAT's practice of collaborative reformulation aims to reflect and understand what each service user brings to therapy, including their cultural assumptions and formation".

Within this guide, we aim to stay true to CAT's radically social view of the self, whilst also pushing our collective zone of proximal development (ZPD, Vygotsky, 1978), a little further into the consideration of issues of power, equality, and diversity in CAT. We hope that the explicit inclusion of service user voice within this book will help to stretch our ability to think critically in relation to these crucial issues.

A note on diagnosis

We acknowledge that the concept of diagnosis in mental health can be a contentious issue. On the one hand, there are many valid critiques of the application of the medical model of health and illness to the concept of psychological well-being. On the other, many people can experience the process of receiving a diagnosis to be one of relief and validation. CAT's approach has largely been a transdiagnostic one, aiming to focus more on the relational origin and maintenance of 'problematic' patterns (survival strategies) and reciprocal roles, rather than on mental health 'symptoms' and 'labels'. Despite this, there have been attempts to make sense of diagnostic concepts and presentations using CAT thinking – for example what is commonly referred to as 'borderline personality disorder' (The Multiple Self States Model; Ryle, 1997).

It feels hugely important to acknowledge the psychological harm that terminology can cause, as well as the comfort it can bring. With this in mind, we strive to explore and describe key CAT concepts and processes through a lens that is trauma informed, respecting the strategies that people develop in order to survive and holding in mind that there is no one truth when it comes to infinitely varied human experience.

The flexibility of the model

As therapists, we are perhaps more effective in our practice when we are working within a model that broadly aligns with our preferences, values and personalities. Undoubtedly, we also recognise the need for the therapist to adapt their approach to meet the service user's needs as much as possible. CAT combines a strong relational frame with the space and freedom for service user and therapist to metaphorically 'meet each other where they need to'. Our belief in the CAT model has stood the test of time, and as a creative, flexible approach, we believe that CAT will too. Nevertheless, we should not rest on our laurels – we live in an ever-changing world, and CAT must continue to evolve and adapt if it hopes to truly meet the needs of those it serves.

The word 'unprecedented' has been overused in recent years – but perhaps little else can describe the devastating impact of the coronavirus pandemic on our communities. We found ourselves very quickly needing to change the way we worked in order to continue supporting those amongst us who were most vulnerable. Necessity was the mother of invention as we saw the widespread adoption of remote working practices and online therapy sessions. Whilst these ways of relating cannot be compared with face-to-face interactions, they have perhaps allowed us to begin to think differently about what had been assumed, with good reason, to be the 'givens' of talking therapies. For many receiving (and offering) therapy, online sessions may not be a preference, but for others, this option opened doors that may have until now been mostly closed. For us, this raises the more general question of how authentically we are able to offer choice within the work that we do – how much are we *really* willing and able to meet our service users where they need to be met (both literally and figuratively)? This will inevitably vary hugely between different services, settings and practitioners; however, we encourage the reader to hold in mind the concepts of choice and flexibility as we journey through this guide together. There is no one set way for a practitioner to offer and deliver CAT. Our narrative is a guide to show ways in which it 'can be done', yet we urge you to consider your own style, values and preferred psychological theories as you develop your skills within CAT. This will then sit hand in hand with the flexibility, creativity and choice that you can offer to the service user.

What to expect

Whilst introducing you to the key terms and concepts of CAT, this book will also provide current guidance and considerations in relation to the different 'parts' of the CAT contract. We will focus on therapy from a one-to-one perspective, rather than attending to the wider organisational uses of CAT that have developed in more recent years. First and foremost, when therapists are training in CAT, learning the 'how-to' of practising CAT as a direct approach is paramount, and it can take time and effort to feel skilled in each area. Each chapter will consider a specific element of CAT, within the structure of the therapy, from assessment through to saying goodbye. It is hoped that each chapter can stand alone, for you to read as and when you are ready, or as part of a wider whole, leading you stage by stage through the therapeutic approach.

Karen and Andrew will also have space to reflect on their own journey through CAT, and we hope that together, we can provide you with a constructively critical understanding of the model as a whole.

Karen says:

> *I do think it's important our stories are told in the book because you can see the benefits of it and I always recommend it to people, I always say try it because it might just do you good.*

We hope you find the book enjoyable, easy to follow and a useful text to accompany you on your journey with this developing relational approach!

Further Reading

Calvert, R., Kellett, S., & Hagan, T. (2015). Group Cognitive Analytic Therapy for female survivors of childhood sexual abuse. *British Journal of Clinical Psychology*, 54(4), 391–413. https://doi.org/10.1111/bjc.12085

Carradice, A. (2013). 'Five Session CAT' consultancy: Using CAT to guide care planning with people diagnosed with personality disorder within community mental health teams. *Clinical Psychology and Psychotherapy*, 20(4), 359–367. https://doi.org/10.1002/cpp.1812

Clarke, S., Thomas, P., & James, K. (2013). Cognitive Analytic Therapy for personality disorder: Randomised control trial. *British Journal of Psychiatry*, 202, 129–134. https://doi.org/10.1192/bjp.bp.112.108670

Denman, C. (2001). Cognitive Analytic Therapy. *Advances in Psychiatric Treatment*, 7, 243–256. https://doi.org/10.1192/apt.7.4.243

Felitti, V. J., Anda, R. F., Nordenberg, D., Williamson, D. F., Spitz, A. M., Edwards, V., Koss, M. P., & Marks, J. S. (1998). Relationship of childhood abuse and household dysfunction to many of the leading causes of death in adults. The Adverse Childhood Experiences (ACE) study. *American Journal of Preventive Medicine*, 14(4), 245–258. https://doi.org/10.1016/s0749-3797(98)00017-8

Feltham, C. & Horton, I. (2012). *Handbook of Counselling and Psychotherapy*. (3rd Ed). Sage.

Fosbury, J. A., Bosley, C. M., Ryle, A., Sonksen, P. H., & Judd, S. L. (1997). A trial of Cognitive Analytic Therapy in poorly controlled type 1 patients. *Diabetes Care*, 20, 959–964. https://doi.org/10.2337/diacare.20.6.959

Johnstone, L., Boyle, M., Cromby, J., Dillon, J., Harper, D., Kinderman, P., Longden, E., Pilgrim, D., & Read, J. (2018). *The Power Threat Meaning Framework: Towards the Identification of Patterns in Emotional Distress, Unusual Experiences and Troubled or Troubling Behaviour, as an Alternative to Functional Psychiatric Diagnosis*. British Psychological Society.

Kellett, S., et al. (2019). Delivering cognitive analytic consultancy to community mental health teams: Initial practice-based evidence from a multi site evaluation. *Psychology and Psychotherapy: Theory, Research and Practice*, 93, 429–455. https://doi.org/10.1111/papt.12221

Kelly, G. A. (1955). *The Psychology of Personal Constructs. Volume 1: A theory of personality*. Norton.

Leiman, M. (1970). The development of Cognitive Analytic Therapy. *International Journal of Short-Term Psychotherapy*, 9, 67–81.

Marriott, M. & Kellett, S. (2009). Evaluating a Cognitive Analytic Therapy service: Practice-based outcomes and comparisons with person-centred and cognitive behavioural therapies. *Psychology and Psychotherapy Theory Research and Practice*, 82(1), 57–72. https://doi.org/10.1248/147608308X336100

Ougrin, D., Zundel, T., Ng, A., Banarsee, R., Bottle, A., & Taylor, E. (2011). Trial of Therapeutic Assessment in London: randomised controlled trial of Therapeutic Assessment versus standard psychosocial assessment in adolescents presenting with self-harm. *Archives of Disease in Childhood*, 96(2), 148–153. https://doi.org/10.1136/adc.2010.188755

Ryle, A. (1985). Cognitive theory, object relations and the self. *British Journal of Medical Psychology*, 58(1), 1–7.

Ryle, A. (Ed.). (1995). *Cognitive Analytic Therapy: Developments in Theory and Practice*. John Wiley & Sons Ltd.

Ryle, A. (1997). *Cognitive Analytic Therapy and Borderline Personality Disorder: The Model and the Method*. John Wiley & Sons Ltd.

Ryle, A. & Kerr, I. (2002). *Introducing Cognitive Analytic Therapy. Principles and Practice*. Wiley.

Ryle, A., Kellett, S., Hepple, J. et al. (2014). Cognitive Analytic Therapy at 30. *Advances in Psychiatric Treatment*, 20(4), 258–268. https://doi.org/10.1192/apt.bp.113.011817

Treasure, J. & Ward, A. (1999). Cognitive Analytic Therapy in the treatment of anorexia nervosa. *Clinical Psychology and Psychotherapy*, 4(1), 62–71. https://doi.org/10.1002/(SICI)1099-0879(199703)4:1%3C62::AID-CPP114%3E3.0.CO;2-Y

Vygotsky, L. S. (1978). *Mind in Society: The Development of Higher Psychological Processes*. Harvard University Press.

Walsh, S. (1996). Adapting Cognitive Analytic Therapy to make sense of psychologically harmful work environments. *British Journal of Medical Psychology*, 69(1), 3–20. https://doi.org/10.1111/j.2044-8341.1996.tb01846.x

Walsh, S. (2019). 'Infamy, infamy, they've all got it in for me'. Exits in Organisationally Informed CAT Supervision. *Reformulation*, Summer, 6–8.

Winnicott, D. W. (1965). *The Maturational Processes and the Facilitating Environment.* International Universities Press.

2   Service user perspectives

Introduction

As mentioned in the first chapter, Karen and Andrew have consented to share their own stories, their experiences of CAT, the CAT tools and their perspectives on the different parts of the model. Karen's and Andrew's viewpoints will be interwoven throughout the book, so you can see first-hand the impact that CAT can have from a personal perspective. We have had a number of conversations with Karen and Andrew throughout the development of the book and wanted them to feel able to share honestly, openly and critically their views of the model. Both Karen and Andrew have chosen to use their real names, and in doing so, were eager to ensure that the reality of CAT was communicated within the book. We have, however, chosen not to refer by name to anyone else who is mentioned in their stories, in order to preserve their anonymity. Additionally, their therapists have provided consent for the inclusion of the therapy tools within this text. Karen has also written her own book, sharing her experience of bipolar disorder, entitled *Searching for Better Days: Learning to Manage my Bipolar Brain* (Manton, 2017). In this chapter, we hand over to Karen and Andrew to share with you their early life experiences and what led them to engage in a contract of CAT. It should be noted that their stories contain elements which some readers may find distressing, such as firsthand experiences of domestic violence and suicide attempts.

Karen's experience

As I reflect on my CAT, I am quite surprised to see that this took place just over ten years ago. It seems far more recent than that. I recall at the time of requesting therapy that I was having difficulties coming to terms with events that had taken place throughout my childhood. I became aware that every time I talked to my husband about those years, I couldn't hold back the tears.

I was raised an only child, with my parents, despite having five half-siblings. My dad was a heavy drinker and sadly this would often lead to domestic violence with my mam, who was always the victim. Mam had insecurities and because of this she would often want to be out socialising with him. This would

DOI: 10.4324/9781003308256-2

often result in me being handed over to my nana to be looked after, or on occasion left alone as a very young child, with a neighbour popping in to check on my safety. Sadly, this was quite common in the 1970s.

At the age of 43 years, these memories were starting to affect me, and I knew I needed to address them. I mentioned this to my consultant, and he suggested CAT. I wasn't sure what this was about, but I was prepared to embark on anything that might help me to come to terms with my past.

My referral for CAT mentioned my history of bipolar disorder and the fact that in recent months I had wanted psychological therapy to address residual anxiety, low self-esteem and traumatic memories. It described how I had been in remission on medication since 2002 and how I continued to have outpatient follow-up because of the severity of previous episodes, which included regular detention under the Mental Health Act and prolonged hospitalisation. It also mentioned how my earlier episodes did seem to be precipitated by life events – relationship difficulties and marital breakdown. I was presently in a stable relationship which I had benefitted from.

It wasn't long before I was invited to my first appointment to meet with my therapist. To my relief she appeared to be a very pleasant, caring young lady who I would have no trouble relating to. After our initial conversation I was asked to complete some questionnaires; this was to give the therapist an understanding of my present state of mind. We discussed what I hoped to get from my therapy, and I explained how I wanted to come to terms with my past events.

Over the course of the next four weeks, she would listen intently as I talked about my life at present, my relationship with my husband, my children and my mam. She needed to get an understanding of me, what my thoughts and feelings were and how my past was contributing to my present. We talked at great length about my childhood, the positives and the negatives.

The therapist then drew a map and based on the information I was giving her, she titled it with:
'Target problem': "I find it difficult to deal with pressure from others – Unable to be assertive/too aggressive/fear of breakdown."
Underneath was:
Striving (perfect) to Pressured
(Trying to be the perfect mother/wife/daughter) leading to
Dependency/Demanding/Merging to Strangulated/Stifled
(My needs not met, no one looking after me) leading to
Criticising/Neglecting to Uncared for/Not listened to/Angry
And in the centre of all of this was
Not cared for

The map was a summary of my thoughts and feelings following all those years of traumatic memories.
As the therapist worked on the map, I wasn't aware of how significant this would be, not until we reached the end of my therapy.

At session 4, my therapist wrote a letter to me and asked me to read it to see if she had gained a clear understanding of my life and my hopes for therapy. As I read the letter it was clear she had certainly understood me, and in a way that maybe I wasn't understanding myself.

It was in this letter that she highlighted how my childhood (and often being left alone or 'palmed off' to my nana) had left me feeling neglected. Hence the map shows neglecting to neglected/uncared for. It was mentioned how my fiery temperament seemed to follow that of my dad's, and she wondered if my automatic aggressive response to conflict came from my childhood, as this seemed to be the way with my parents.

My therapist mentioned how part of my reason for coming to therapy was to deal with issues from my past, so that I did not take out my issues on my mam, who was now in her 80s. She explained how our early relationship had become enmeshed and that my mam's dependence on me had meant that in fact I had become the parent and, therefore, I was not being looked after in the way that I should have been at such a young age.

We understood how this had continued into my later life, when I found it difficult to detach from my mam; despite being in my first marriage; there was very little time for privacy, as my mam had visited almost every night. I was now resenting this and feeling 'strangulated' – I was feeling that everyone had been leaning on me which was coupled with the fact that I was very demanding of myself. The map shows dependency/demanding/merging to strangulated and stifled.

The letter then went on to describe how I had several hospital admissions when I was married to my first husband and that it was not a good experience. It perhaps was linked to the criticising/neglecting reciprocal role. I hadn't found staff to be caring and felt they were judgmental of me. My therapist wondered if I had hoped for the care that I did not seem to be getting from anyone else. I had felt there was no support in my first marriage, and I often felt that I was in/occupying the mother role in relation to my husband. I was regularly unwell and showed symptoms of my bipolar illness every two years. I felt that he had pressured me into a termination just before our marriage, and despite going on to have two beautiful children together, an affair on his part did contribute to breaking up the marriage.

It was at this point that my therapist pointed out how it was interesting to see that my last hospital admission was in 2002, and how my mental health had improved since meeting my future husband in 2003. She did suggest that I had an underlying fear of ever losing him and maybe that was the reason I strived to be the 'perfect' wife. She shared that despite heated debates when I didn't feel listened to, overall, my husband appeared to give me the support and care that was perhaps missing as a child, and that I didn't perhaps get from my first marriage; hence the reason why I have now remained well.

At this point my therapist discussed in the letter how I was trying to exit from dependency and strangulation and to find more space for myself and how learning assertiveness skills would help in this area. She was also aware that I constantly strive for perfection, which may have come from my father always wanting me to achieve 100 per cent, but how this has continued into my adult life with me wanting the perfect home. It was pointed out that my target problem was about the difficulty I had in dealing with pressure from others, which resulted in my aggression leading to further conflict. We needed to look at ways of helping me to manage pressure/demands and stress without being aggressive, feeling guilty or not feeling perfect.

To summarise her letter, my therapist stated that assertiveness skills would help me; finding ways to say no, doing things on my terms and finding a middle ground. Detaching a little and finding space to relax and be myself would also help. Also talking to my husband to let him know my needs so that I felt that I was being listened to, if done in an assertive manner, could help. It was pointed out that I may encounter issues in therapy; for instance, if I strived to be the perfect patient, I may feel angry if I took something the therapist said as a criticism or I may also become over attached to the therapy and feel neglected at the end. These were all things we both needed to be mindful of and which we could deal with if and when they arose.

As the letter ended it was suggested at week 4, that we meet for 16 sessions overall.

I was amazed at how the therapist completely understood me. Already I was starting to see how the therapy was making me question myself and see things from a different angle. I was determined to make this work for me.

Every week I ensured I turned up on time for my therapy and I felt fully engaged with it. I knew that it wasn't going to be an easy ride but that it was necessary to help me move forward with my life.

Over the weeks that followed I completed more questionnaires, which monitored my mental state. I completely understood the reasons for this as I know my therapist would want to ensure that I was coping with the therapy and of course the last thing she would have wanted is for this to have an adverse effect on my mental illness.

I was often given tasks to complete to enable my growth. I recall one week it was suggested that perhaps I write a letter to my mum, requesting to know why certain things had happened over the years, resulting in making me feel neglected. It was suggested that I express my feelings on paper to see if this release would help me to better understand my feelings. The letter was intended to be just for my own reading. At my appointment the following week, my therapist asked if I had managed to accomplish this. However, she was quite taken aback when I shared that instead of writing the letter, I had visited mam to discuss this with her. This had taken place in a very calm and caring manner, and I was delighted to report that it had really helped me. It had allowed me not only to express the hurt that I had felt but to gain an understanding of why this had happened, an acknowledgement from mam that it hadn't been appropriate, and that looking back things should have been done very differently. This had given me some closure from mam and a greater understanding of her situation at the time. I felt in many ways this did help to heal an old wound. My therapist was delighted at the hard work that had been put into this and that I had found it so beneficial.

When we reached the end of our 16 sessions my therapist wrote a therapeutic goodbye letter to me for the context of CAT. The letter summarised the things shared, what we had learned and the exits that I had made. It was at this point we returned to the map and a new map was produced.

My healthy map showed the heading as: 'I can deal with pressure from others by being assertive, keeping some distance and not feeling guilty about it'.

Underneath now read:

Good enough
Relaxed
Unpressured
(Don't have to be the perfect mother/wife/daughter) leading to
Distancing/Assertive to Free/Independent no guilt
(Look after self/Gain care from own family) leading to
Caring/Kind (to self) Cared for
(Think about/look after myself)

My therapist had then added notes to the original map, showing how I had achieved this, which included distancing myself, being assertive, saying no and things being managed more on my terms. My perfection became learning to accept 'Good Enough' – things don't have to be perfect. I don't have to be perfect. My criticising became relaxing 'me time', which all enabled me to remain calm whilst being assertive.

As I looked at the maps, I was amazed that those were the issues that I had. Many will ask how I had made those changes and if I'm entirely honest, even I'm not sure of that. I just know it was a slow process and a lot of hard work. I was amazed that I had managed to detach myself from my mam, obviously being there when she needed me, but not feeling the pressure and the guilt that I had always endured. If mam now needed something from me, I knew it was acceptable to do this on my terms, when I had the time, which enabled the pressure to subside.

My therapist felt that I had been very strong to learn to stand my ground, to keep a distance, but at the same time to retain the loving relationship, which was so important to me. I accepted that I needed to relax without the feeling of guilt. The only issue which we agreed still needed some work was learning to control my anger, which had got better but was still a work in progress.

My therapeutic goodbye letter acknowledged the hard work that I had put into my CAT, and the therapist hoped that I would continue to reap the rewards of this. As my therapy ended, it was suggested that we meet up eight weeks later, to see how things were going. At this point I had also written a closure letter describing my experience of CAT. I am pleased to say that we met later and that I managed my therapy closure in a very positive manner.

Ten years later I can reflect on my therapy and know that it helped me to become a much happier version of myself. It was certainly a roller-coaster of emotions, and many weeks I felt quite drained from the tears that I shed, in acknowledging my past. However, I wasn't deterred by this as I knew it was never going to be an easy road. I must be honest and say there is nothing that I would have changed about any part of my CAT. I felt blessed to have found a therapist that I could connect with. She wasn't a therapist who would agree with all my views, but she would listen to me and then encourage me to look at something from a different angle, enabling me to question my thoughts.

Even today I still remind myself that I don't need to be perfect, and I still hear my therapist's voice reminding me of 'Good Enough'. As the years have passed, I am aware that I still do have a temper, but more importantly I have learned how to control this, especially in situations where it certainly would not be warranted.

I am so grateful that my therapy allowed me to heal old wounds with my mam, especially as she went on to develop vascular dementia and Alzheimer's disease. My therapy gave me the strength to make the right decisions for my mam's care and to speak up when things were not quite right. Sadly, mam passed away in February 2020, but I was with her to the very end and knew she passed away knowing that we both worshipped each other.

My experience of CAT was just brilliant, and my advice would be, if you are prepared to work at it and deal with those often-uncomfortable emotions, it can be so beneficial. In fact, I would go as far to say it can be life changing.

'Life is a journey and CAT enables you to continue on that journey'.

Andrew's experience

My name is Andrew; I'm 50, married, with two lovely kids. I have suffered with depression since my early teens. This is my journey:

You will have to bear with me I'm afraid, my memory is not great so some of what I will write might not have even happened and I sure as hell won't be putting any dates or exact ages as I just plain don't know.

The depression came about because of an accident, not to me but to my father. We jokingly say that he fell off the back off a lorry; actually, he was leaning against a support on the back of a wagon when it collapsed, he and a fellow worker fell, and my dad was left with a fractured skull, an altered personality and never worked again. I can't remember exactly how I was told; I think it was by my friend's mother and I vaguely remember having to stay with them for a few days.

I do remember walking into the living room when my dad got out of hospital; I was warned to be gentle as he was quite fragile. He had two black eyes and looked very frail. At the age I was, your dad is superman! He wasn't supposed to be like this. I seem to remember vowing that I would have to be the man of the house. I say dad never worked again; he did work for a little while because he had another accident at work when he cut his head open!

As I said, I believed I needed to be the man of the house, a role I was not ready for, although no one else had any expectations of me. There is something else that preyed on my mind at this time. When my dad was 16 his father died, I was paranoid that history was going to repeat itself, especially given how ill my dad was. I remember being very relieved when I turned 17; we had cheated history.

When I left school, I went to Art College to do my BTec in fashion. I had been 'well built' for most of senior school, [but] I decided I was fat, so pretty much stopped eating. I'm not going to say I had anorexia, but it was pretty close. I went from a 38″ waist to about a 24″ at my worst, I collapsed in a bathroom in Paris on a college trip, and I wasn't well. It got to the point where it hurt more to eat than it did to not eat. I have a picture of me during that time, wearing a baggy jumper to hide my body; I look like I could snap if I bent over.

After college I started working in the fashion industry, probably one of the most stressful environments to work in. I lasted about 15 years with various episodes of the black dog (depression), but I still didn't know what it was, I had talked about suicide with my then girlfriend (now wife), but I thought that was normal! Eventually the first glimpse into what was actually happening to me came about. We were told the company I was working for wanted us all to move to Leicester as that was closer to head office; this was never an option for me as my wife worked here, we had just had a baby, and moved to a new house we loved. Of course, the alternative was redundancy. I became ill, I would sleep up to 22 hours a day, I became dehydrated as I couldn't stay awake long enough to drink. I kept going back to the doctors, who kept sending me for tests, diabetes, thyroid, all sorts. I asked if it could be stress related. He then asked if I was stressed. I explained that I was being made redundant; we had just had a baby and moved into a house that was about twice the mortgage of our previous home (in our previous house we had been broken into four times over two years, including twice in one week). After three months on the sick, the doctor decided I was ill because I was overweight.

After I left the fashion industry I started a business making clothes and soft furnishings [and] my wife went back to work full-time. I also started a part-time degree in textiles. This had become a pattern for me: take too much on so I would fail; this would then prove to me how useless I felt, how much of a failure I was, and why I was not worth knowing or loving.

Eventually of course it all came to a head!

My wife had to go to Austria with work and it would be over a weekend. It would have been almost impossible for her to come home, so her company paid for me to meet her in Salzburg for the weekend. We had a long chat as things had not been great between us for a while, we decided I needed to go and see a different doctor and tell him what was going on. I flew back home, and my wife went back to work. I didn't eat while she was away, I was punishing myself, food felt like the one thing I had control over. I sat one night, kids in bed, and took every pill and quite a lot of whiskey I could find and sat back, feeling calm for the first time in years. This was it, my time to clock out.

Of course, it suddenly struck me that it would be my kids that would find me, I was a horrible person, but I couldn't do that to them! I took myself to the toilet and made myself throw up until I had nothing left then stayed up all night in case I fell asleep and didn't wake up. It's funny, but shortly after this we had a party for my daughter's birthday, and lots of people commented on how well I looked! I had shaved my head as my hair was falling out; I had a haunted look in my eyes.

We went to the doctors and told him how I felt; he asked my wife if I ever hit her or the kids. I was horrified at the time, but I can see he was asking all the right questions. My life was in freefall, and I had absolutely no control. I was prescribed anti-depressants, sent home and told to wait for the crisis team. They arrived at our house not long after us, two ladies, one went and spoke to my wife, and the other sat and let me talk. They visited a couple of times until I was relatively stable. I'm not sure if it was a complete nervous breakdown, but it's as close as I ever want to be.

The doctor recommended 'Mind' (a mental health charity) to me; they were great and dug into what was causing the depression as well as giving me coping strategies. The first time I went there I felt like the world was in colour and not the black and white I had seen it [in] for years. I went on to see Mind several times after that as the depression would find its way back.

I finally felt strong enough to ask the doctor if I could have some counselling, which he arranged. I remember sitting in the waiting room with my wife, everyone had various nervous twitches, no one would give eye contact, and when you caught a glimpse of their eyes, it was terrifying, I wondered what they saw when they looked at me; for sure I had the same.

I felt terrible about the amount of medication I was on, largest dosage of anti-depressants plus another type to help me sleep, all of this just to help me feel 'normal'. I had told my therapist that this felt like the last chance for me as I couldn't go on feeling the way I was; I realise how melodramatic that was now, but I meant it at the time. I think I realised that this might work, and I was ready for it too; when the therapist asked what I wanted, previously when asked I would say that I just wanted to be like everyone else, this time I said I just wanted to be comfortable being me! I can see now what a huge shift that statement was.

I had a full course of CAT, which I feel gave me the tools to finally get to grips with my issues. CAT gave me a road map, or as I refer to it, an internal sat-nav. If you are wondering, the voice of that sat-nav is still my therapist's voice. I don't remember a lot of the details of each session, but I do recall them being hard work. I almost didn't turn up for my second session, and every time I had a session, the rest of the day would be written off, I was so drained. I found my letter again fairly recently, and it's actually really hard to put myself back in that mindset. CAT for me was the real beginning of the road to recovery. As helpful and necessary as all my other therapies were pre-CAT, it was only when I started that everything clicked into place. Up until that point, we had been 'firefighting'.

I can say now that this therapy saved my life, has allowed me to live a more comfortable existence, and to look forward to the future, a future I now see myself in. I am still learning about myself and my mental health but everything I learn has followed on from CAT. I used to think I was stupid because here I was in my fifties, just figuring things out. In truth, CAT gave me the space and the tools to learn these things. Now I purely think of it as a journey I needed to take.

I'd like to say that that was the end of my journey; I had hit rock bottom and over the course of about seven years, I had crawled my way out of it, from near death and self-harm to loving life. Growing up I could never see myself growing old; I was sure I would be dead by 37! I started to become ill again a few years ago and after a lot of tests I was told I had ankylosing spondylitis (a form of arthritis that predominantly affects the sacroiliac joint), but the medication was often worse than the illness. Earlier this year, my diagnosis was changed to fibromyalgia, which can apparently be brought on by depression. I have been unable to work over the last few years due to my condition.

For people who don't know what fibromyalgia is, it's basically constant pain, generally all over. I can't walk far, I have no upper body strength anymore, can't lift, can't even put my arms above my head without pain. So of course, the depression keeps rearing its ugly head. Thankfully, I now have the tools to stop me sliding to the bottom of the pit. I still receive counselling, periodically, when needed but my mental health is the best it has ever been, and also the most robust. Recently I have learnt to let go of the past. I've forgiven myself for mistakes I've made; it has made a huge impact on my life, and it all started with CAT. Due to my health issues, I am on a lot of medication and will be for life. I am still on anti-depressants, but it no longer bothers me. I realise that it's just what I need to keep me well.

Thank you for getting this far, I know I tend to ramble and have probably missed out so much, but there you go!

Conclusion

We are indebted to Karen and Andrew for their openness, candidness and commitment within this book. To share with you their perspectives on CAT in more detail, we met with them for a day, to have conversations about each of the different stages of CAT and what they remember about the process. These conversations were recorded and transcribed, so that we can use their voices firsthand throughout the book.

References

Manton, K. (2017). *Searching for Brighter Days: Learning to Manage My Bipolar Brain.* Trigger.

3 Principles of Cognitive Analytic Therapy

Introduction

Before we explore the 'how-to' of the different parts of CAT, it is important to understand further some of the main principles that underpin the approach. In particular, we explore the concepts embedded within CAT from a C (cognitive) and A (analytic) perspective and provide examples of how their theories are used within the CAT model. Further focus is then given to the four Rs in CAT, namely, reformulation, recognition, revision and relationship. As a means to consider the 'how-to' of structuring a CAT contract, we then provide detail as to what in general a contract to 16 sessions would look like.

The beginnings of CAT

Qualifying in medicine in 1949, Tony Ryle began as a GP in North London, which coincided with the inception of the NHS, and as we shall see, he aligned himself closely with the principles of the new health service. During his early years in general practice, Ryle became increasingly interested in what his service users were telling him about their emotional, as well as their physical problems. This led him to conduct epidemiological research on the prevalence and origins of common psychological difficulties (by age, gender and social class) within his own practice population (Association for Cognitive Analytic Therapy, ACAT, 2016). His socialist and egalitarian principles influenced the development of some of CAT's key features; recognising the high prevalence of untreated psychological difficulties in the population he was serving, he was naturally drawn to the creation of a practical and time-limited therapy (Ryle et al., 2014).

In the mid-1960s Ryle began working within a University Health Service (ACAT, 2016). His interest in psychological issues had evolved throughout his years in general practice, and his role at the university allowed him both to pursue research, using Kelly's (1955) repertory grid techniques, whilst also to work clinically with university students. Although not formally trained in psychotherapy, Ryle, during this time, was supervised by a psychoanalyst (Ryle et al., 2014). Ryle found the concepts of transference and countertransference

DOI: 10.4324/9781003308256-3

(the feelings that emerge between therapists and service users) to be helpful and, influenced by object relations theory, he began to consider how early relationships between parent and child are internalised. Ryle observed that the multitude of different psychotherapies, each with their own distinct underpinning theories and terminology, meant that it was difficult for practitioners from different schools of thought to communicate meaningfully with one another. Whilst being drawn to psychoanalytic thought and concepts, and seeing their use in clinical practice, he also at times struggled to make sense of psychoanalytic writings. In seeking to create a 'common language for the psychotherapies', Ryle found himself integrating ideas from psychoanalytic thought with his own observations from clinical practice, particularly from his use of Kelly's (1955) repertory grid techniques (a method of understanding the ways in which someone gives meaning to their experiences). Through his analysis of case notes from completed psychotherapies, Ryle was able to identify three broad categories of unhelpful yet unrevised patterns of relating to themselves and others that service users frequently appeared to become caught up in. The resultant traps, snags and dilemmas (see Chapter 5 for definitions of these concepts), as we now know them, drew upon understandings from behavioural, psychoanalytic and personal construct theories. Ryle subsequently found that in identifying and collaboratively naming someone's problematic 'procedures', as they came to be known (essentially, problematic patterns of thinking, behaving and relating), it became more possible to recognise them in action and, consequently, to revise them.

He formally proposed CAT as a psychotherapy in the mid-1980s, attempting to restate psychoanalytic concepts in less mystifying and more practical terms. The model has been refined and developed over the decades since its inception, however, it has remained true to the principles upon which it was based (e.g., integration at the level of theory, a common language for the psychotherapies and the provision of an accessible and time-limited therapy that can be adapted to meet the needs of the service user).

The contribution of the C

Whilst the contributions of cognitive and behavioural theory and practice in CAT may not be as explicitly named within the development of the model, their influence upon its form and structure are plain to see. As Ryle et al. (2014) have pointed out, the therapeutic technique in CAT has much in common with cognitive behavioural approaches – both of which emphasise the development of a collaborative working relationship with the service user and a shared descriptive formulation of their current difficulties.

The cognitive behavioural approach, in contrast to psychodynamic ways of working, takes care to express concepts in operational terms and ensures that all aspects of therapy are made explicit to the service user. This therapeutic 'transparency' has much in common with CAT and goes some way to address the power imbalances that are inherent in the therapeutic relationship and in modalities where this may not be as explicit. In addition to this, CBT's emphasis on goal setting, self-monitoring, homework and becoming one's own therapist is clearly mirrored in CAT.

The influence of CBT upon CAT does not end at the level of structure and process; it can also be observed to some degree in the content of their overlapping theoretical concepts. Beck's application of cognitive approaches to depression in 1967 emphasised the importance of unhelpful thinking styles and behaviours, in the maintenance of low mood. Considering these key theoretical components, we see the influence of CBT on CAT, in particular within CAT's concept of 'traps', that is, vicious cycles of related thoughts, feelings and behaviours which are self-defeating but remain unrevised. Traps are ultimately patterns within which a negative belief influences behaviour in such a way that the consequences of the behaviour tend to either maintain the difficulty or appear to confirm the original belief. Depressed thinking, avoidance and social isolation (both of which are broadly anxiety-based), and low self-esteem traps could all be thought of as mini-cross-sectional CBT maintenance formulations (comprising associated *emotions, bodily sensations, thoughts* and *behaviours*) of these common presenting difficulties. For example, the avoidance trap begins with the statements "I feel anxious and not very confident about certain situations – when I go into these situations I feel more anxious"; this describes the *emotions* that someone may experience and hints at possible cognitions or *beliefs* about the self in terms of not feeling very confident. The trap goes on to state that "avoiding these situations makes me feel better, so I stop trying to face them" – here we can clearly see the influence of behaviourism in terms of the concept of negative reinforcement; an unpleasant *bodily sensation* (i.e., anxiety) is removed by avoiding these situations; hence the *behaviour* becomes negatively reinforced (in other words, we are more likely to do the thing that brought us the sense of relief again in the future). Unfortunately, however, the behaviour also has some unintended consequences: the trap concludes by stating "my life becomes more limited, and I feel more anxious and less confident". This hints at the processes thought to underlie the maintenance of anxiety difficulties, from a CBT perspective – avoiding situations which trigger unpleasant emotions and bodily sensations may bring short-term relief; however, as the need to employ these avoidance strategies becomes more entrenched, not only does life become more limited (with fewer opportunities for potentially enjoyable activities), but we erroneously conclude that the only reason something bad didn't happen was that we employed a 'safety behaviour' – in this case, avoidance. In other words, we rob ourselves of the opportunity to learn that it might have been OK/we might have been able to cope, and this keeps us stuck in the cycle of anxiety and avoidance.

Certain CBT principles such as a focus on symptoms, disorder-specific conceptualisations and manualised treatments do not bear much resemblance to CAT. Yet, as Denman (2001) points out, those working within the schema focussed tradition of CBT (Young, 1990) are likely to adopt a more similar style of bespoke case conceptualisation to CAT practitioners and will find much that is similar between the two approaches. Schema therapy makes sense of entrenched and problematic ways of relating to self and others through the concept of 'early maladaptive schemas' – pervasive patterns that are developed during early life with key caregivers as a way of coping with the circumstances that a person finds themselves in. Like CAT, this approach also makes explicit use of the therapeutic relationship in working through these patterns.

The contribution of the A

The concepts which CAT has developed from psychoanalytic thinking are immensely useful in making sense of relational experiences and patterns; however, those new to CAT can often feel mystified by some of the terminology that is associated with these analytic theories. Here we aim to navigate through these ideas with just the lightest of touches; this is in no way to diminish the vast contribution of psychoanalytic ideas to our understanding of the development of the self and of the practice of psychotherapy, but rather to keep us true to our aims of providing an accessible guide for the reader. We will make links to the CAT concepts that these ideas underpin here; however, for a more detailed explanation of the key CAT terms and ideas, see Chapter 5.

The contributions of object relations theory

Object relations theory (Fairburn, 1954) introduces us to the idea that we develop an *internal sense (or template)* of key people, and our relationships with them, in our lives from a young age. These internalised representations also impact upon how we relate to and view ourselves. It is this idea that forms the basis for the concept of 'reciprocal roles' within CAT, something we shall return to repeatedly in the coming chapters. There might be lots of things that make up our internal sense of, say, our mother or father. Memories of things that have happened, things they said, how they made us feel. We also know that our internal representations of someone can never be an exact replica of that person. We might remember certain things but not others. Our internal sense of that key person might be based partly on things other people have told us about them; it will inevitably also be skewed by all the things we *didn't* know about them. So, our representations are just that: representations. Despite this, they are very powerful, and as we shall see, can form a lens through which we see ourselves, the world and others.

In the complex world we live in, our brains must find efficient ways to understand and organise the vast amount of information we are subject to; this involves also being able to make predictions about what we can expect from others and when this may pose a threat. This is potentially a useful shortcut to help us survive; for example, if Dad always becomes argumentative when he's drunk, I quickly learn that when he's been drinking, I keep out of his way. Unfortunately, though, once I'm grown up, anything that reminds me of my internal sense of 'drunk Dad' might result in me withdrawing from whomever or whatever has triggered this representation, even if it doesn't bear all that much resemblance to the original situation. This isn't my fault; it's just the way my human brain works. Unfortunately, as well as affecting how I relate to others, this internalised representation may also have a negative impact on how I relate *to myself*. For example, I may find that I talk to myself in a bullying or critical way; an *internal* pattern which is inevitably harder to escape from than an external trigger.

All of this sets the scene for some incredibly important relational concepts that psychoanalytic thinking has gifted us with and which form the basis of the idea of reciprocal role procedures. The first of these ideas that we will consider is *transference* (Freud, 1912/1958); this occurs when someone in the here and now unwittingly becomes a 'hook' for us to unconsciously hang one of our internal representations on. Maybe, without my realising it, my supervisor reminds me of my mother, and so triggers my internal representation of her. Our brains are taking these sorts of shortcuts all the time – we are not necessarily fully aware that this is going on – but our brains are essentially trying to save us time, keep us safe or help us understand and process something. So, in a sense we are *transferring* a complex internal representation of one person onto another, and then feeling and acting as though this stuff really *is* about them, when in fact we have just 'hung it on their hook'. In CAT, we might see this if someone has a 'criticising-to-criticised' reciprocal role, perhaps because they grew up with a parent who could be critical of them at times. Transference in CAT terms could consist of someone perceiving another person as relating to them in a critical way, even when this was not the intention.

The concept of *projective identification* (Ogden, 1982) takes this process one step further. When we strongly expect someone to act in a certain way, we can unknowingly nudge the person into doing just this. For example, if we consistently expect others to *ignore our needs* (because this is what happened whilst we were growing up), we might unintentionally behave in ways which allow or invite others into relating to us in this way. Expecting that we will be ignored, we might *never ask for what we need* or *express our preferences*, and, because it is not possible to read minds, this may prevent others from being able to fully understand and respond to our needs. In CAT terms, we might think of this as having invited someone to 'join' the dance of an 'ignoring/neglecting-to-ignored/neglected' reciprocal role procedure.

As well as these internal representations of what we can expect from others, we are also taught certain lessons during childhood about what we should expect from *ourselves*. We may, for example, be taught that certain emotions or behaviours are 'not OK'. Imagine the child who is severely punished by a parent every time they cry. It will become crucial to their survival to suppress or cut off from this type of emotional expression, and even the emotions that link to it. Over time, the child comes to push this part of themselves away, create a wall and 'split' it off from their sense of themselves. This leads us to another way of thinking about the idea of *projection* (Freud, 1911/1958). We may come to feel such contempt and fear towards the prospect of displaying any vulnerability that it is safer to identify oneself as indestructible, maybe even 'identifying with the aggressor' (in this case, the punishing parent) and harshly judge what we perceive as 'weakness' in others. In this way, we are 'projecting' what we can't allow ourselves to feel, or be, onto other people, seeing it in them and denying that it even exists within us. We invite others into this 'dance' with us, unknowingly co-opting them into playing the 'vulnerable' role so that we can stay in the indestructible and safe position. The circle of projective identification is complete when (and if) the other person joins our dance; they have in this moment 'identified' with what we have projected onto them. In CAT terms we might think of this as an 'attacking to vulnerable' reciprocal role in which the child who was punished for showing emotion eventually comes to occupy that attacking position at the top of the role themselves, perceiving and judging others as vulnerable or 'weak', but never connecting with their own feelings of vulnerability.

The concept of projective identification (and by extension, the concepts of reciprocal roles, reciprocal role procedures and enactments, that it gave rise to within the CAT model) is not without the potential for misuse. Whilst there is no doubt that the behaviour and relational styles of others impact upon us, as ours do on others, there is the very real risk that the language of projective identification and reciprocal role enactments can be construed as 'victim blaming' when not used cautiously. It is not uncommon to see service users who, following childhood experiences of abuse, have also become survivors of domestic violence or sexual assault as an adult. In this sense, it may be that until something can be processed more consciously, we are drawn back into situations that feel familiar. However, we find ourselves in dangerous territory if we blindly apply the concept of 'nudging' or 'inviting' others to play a role we expect of them in these cases. Whilst it is possible to acknowledge that we may experience a relational pull towards those who fit the expected internal 'template' that we hold of others, we must be careful at all times not to use language that places blame or responsibility on the survivors of abuse in these descriptions.

The four Rs of CAT

It is well considered within the CAT literature that the phases of CAT consist of three main Rs, those of *reformulation, recognition* and *revision* (Ryle & Kerr, 2020). These will be discussed in turn in the following section, before we consider what we might think of as the all-important fourth R in CAT – the *relationship*. In theory, the ordering of these Rs sounds naturally linear, with the service user and therapist working on a shared understanding of the difficulties towards the start of the therapy contract (reformulation), to the therapist and service user noticing patterns both in the therapy and outside of sessions (recognition), and then the service user finding ways of stepping out of the problematic patterns through exits (revision). In practice, therapy is rarely (if ever!) this simple. From experience, we would argue that all of these processes occur in parallel to one another and can each happen at different times throughout the therapeutic process.

Reformulation is always in draft form, as we can never have a 'full' understanding of the service user's presentation, and often it is changed, amended and revised as new information comes to light throughout the developmental process of therapy. Recognition continues all the way through therapy, and beyond, as the service user becomes more self-aware, and some of the patterns that were previously not in their conscious awareness become more noticeable to themselves. This is initially often in hindsight after a situation has occurred, and then in time more so within the moment. Finally, revision too can happen at different stages throughout the contract, from early tentative testing of trying out something new to more mindful challenging of problematic patterns to the more automatic engagement in new, healthier patterns as time goes on.

Figure 3.1 depicts the parallel manner in which each of these Rs occurs throughout therapy. They are not discrete entities (e.g., one does not stop as another starts); they are fluid events that continue to occur interchangeably throughout the contract of therapy.

In addition to the three Rs highlighted within the CAT literature, a focus is perhaps most importantly given to the collaborative nature of the CAT approach. Considering this, we would therefore suggest the fourth R, that of the (therapeutic) relationship. As understood through the considerations of object relations theory in CAT (Winnicott, 1965), the therapeutic relationship is frequently reflected upon and used to aid change. The therapist may share tentative considerations of when problematic patterns are occurring within the room to help the service user notice their presence and recognise the impact on the relationship. The aim is to support the service user in developing a different understanding of the patterns in light of the new, shared information between the two.

Let us take some time to understand each of these Rs in a little more detail, considering the way in which they are used in therapy, the tools that go alongside them to assist their development and some of the terms you may hear in relation to their use.

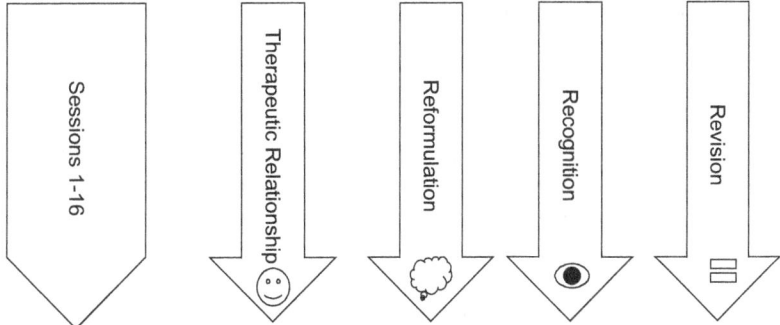

Figure 3.1 The parallel nature of the four Rs.

Reformulation

The process of psychological formulation within therapy is often recognised as a structured approach which is used to understand a service user's distress. Through training others in the use of CAT, we have often been asked the question of what does the 're' mean in reformulation? Originally, Ryle (1991) considered the 're' to be a re-forming of the service user's story. The initial sessions are used within therapy to gain a narrative of the service user's experiences, background history and significant life events that have led to the difficulties they are currently experiencing (we will talk more about CAT assessment a little later). The narrative shared by the service user is then 're-understood' through a CAT lens, through identifying the main positions (or states) a service user finds themselves in, and the repeated patterns within intra- (self) and inter- (others) personal relationships that may maintain the difficulties within the service user's life. It is hoped that the reformulation generates a new understanding of the service user's story, which they find validating, and allows them to begin to appreciate how reciprocal roles have been established throughout their life and how they continue to have an impact.

The reformulation occurs in two main ways in CAT:, through the use of diagrams (also known as a CAT map, or a Sequential Diagrammatic Reformulation) and in prose (through the sharing of the Reformulation Letter) (Ryle & Kerr, 2002). With the reformulation letter generally being shared with the service user around session 4, it can therefore be seen why 'reformulation' is often perceived as an earlier process within the therapeutic contract. Historically, it was felt that the initial three sessions should be used for assessment, with the reformulation letter shared at session 4, and then mapping to begin thereafter (Ryle et al., 2014). Over time, the process has changed, with most CAT practitioners tending to map as early as is feasible with the service user. This serves to begin the development of a shared understanding and to gauge the service user's capacity to reflect and identify any patterns which they have developed as a means of trying to survive. The use of the map and the reformulation letter stay with the service user and therapist throughout the sessions, and should continually be reviewed and reflected upon, to help promote the development of new and increased insight.

Recognition

Quite simply, the second R, for recognition, is what it says on the can. It is the ability in therapy between the service user and therapist to start noticing the problematic patterns and reciprocal roles that have developed and continue to occur for the service user. Here, the overlap between the Rs can be seen, as the process of reformulation begins to assist in early recognition for the service user when patterns are named and identified.

As CAT practitioners, we are often looking out for clues of potential patterns and reciprocal roles with our service users from very early on within the therapeutic contact. The very first meeting with the service user in the waiting room and the gut feeling you experience in relation to them are worth noticing and taking time to stop and reflect upon in supervision. Tentative thinking can even occur prior to the therapy journey itself, for example, through considering information received from referrers and the way in which a service user may be understood by other professionals. Your gathering of information as a thera-pist allows you to enhance your relational thinking and to begin to collate tentative evidence of the patterns of relating the service user engages within. It is understood that if such patterns are occurring with you within the frame of therapy, it is likely that they are happening outside of sessions also.

Upon mapping together within the initial stages of therapy, the CAT prac-titioner will often speak to the service user about the 'observing eye' and add a pictorial drawing of an eye on the top of the map. Here, it is worth discussing with the service user, how the aim of therapy is to begin to develop their own observing eye, through noticing the patterns of relating that are identified on the map, and thus are problematic in maintaining the service user's difficulties. This is known as the process of recognition. However, the means of noticing such problematic procedures is not all the responsibility of the service user. The collaborative nature of the therapy allows for the therapist to have an 'observing eye' also (highlighting patterns to the service user as the therapist may notice them). Throughout therapy, the therapist may take time to 'nudge' the service user outside of their zone of proximal development (ZPD; Vygotsky, 1978), through carefully making reflections upon what may have happened in difficult situations for the service user, in relation to highlighted patterns on the map.

Over the course of therapy, it is hoped that recognition becomes easier for the service user, as they focus more actively on 'noticing' and monitoring the patterns, and overtly discuss them within sessions. We will speak more to the 'how-to' of increasing recognition through monitoring in Chapter 10.

Revision

Revision is a skill that can happen in numerous ways throughout the therapeu-tic contract. From ad hoc changes the service user makes to try out something new to more systematic and agreed modifications the service user attempts, revision is reflected upon, discussed and logged throughout sessions. Revision is often noted as trying out new ways of relating to the self and/or others, in a way of 'exiting' from the service user's target problems (Ryle & Kerr, 2002). Following identification of target problem procedures (the patterns linked to the identified areas of difficulty for the service user; Tanner, 2002) and an intention to monitor or increase the observing eye, the service user uses their new understanding to reconsider their interactions and to adjust their behav-iour whilst also considering the outcome of such a change. For example: through fear of failing an exam and being criticised by their teacher and par-ents, the child learns to strive hard, putting 110 per cent into their revision, which ultimately leads them to burn out prior to the exam, and thus not be well enough to perform at their best. As a result, they are critical of their own sense of self for not succeeding and feel criticised by others for not doing as well as was predicted. As a means of revision, the service user and therapist consider ways to balance and pace their work/rest schedule. In doing so, the service user 'revises' their problematic procedure and learns that they can find a good enough preparation for their exams whilst maintaining their health and wellbeing. In practice, alongside the use of the term 'exit', we have also had service users refer to their revisions as DID: doing it differently!

Relationship

Most psychological therapies highlight the importance of the therapeutic relationship in the course of change within therapy, with some psychologists purporting that the therapeutic relationship alone is an intervention in itself, and that the psychological model is secondary to this (Knobloch-Fedders, 2008). For CAT, the therapeutic relationship is invaluable, and should be central to the practitioner's thinking, both inside and outside of sessions. From the initial meeting, the CAT practitioner aims to create an environment and relationship where the service user feels heard and attended to, forming the basis of a collaborative relationship. The aim within CAT is always to 'be with' the service user rather than 'do to' the service user (Maloney, 2008). In a qualitative study designed to determine nine participants' experiences of CAT, Rayner et al., (2011) found a central theme of 'doing with' the therapist key to making change for the service user. Working jointly with the therapist aided the service user's ability to become more self-aware. Through establishing a collaborative relationship, the therapist is frequently checking in with the service user to ensure the information they share has been understood. This is done through reflecting back the service user's story to them and engaging in therapeutic listening. It is hoped that using such skills will lead the therapist and service user to feel on 'the same wavelength', and for a mutually respectful, equal relationship to be founded (Maloney, 2008). This is particularly beneficial given the natural power imbalance a professional-to-service-user relationship can entail. Instead, CAT aims to minimise an unhealthy role, through recognition that whilst the therapist may be the expert in having psychological knowledge, the service user is the expert in their own life and narrative; thus, joint work is essential to facilitate change.

Alongside the collaborative nature of the therapeutic relationship, the therapist can also 'join the dance' with the service user and end up with them on the map. If a solid foundation within the therapeutic relationship has been built, the therapist may be able to name the dance with the service user, thus aiming to recognise problematic patterns when they are occurring between the two. Similarly, at times in which a therapeutic rupture may occur or where the relationship may break down (for example, if a therapist is off sick and the service user experiences this as a rejection, and subsequently misses the following session), the therapist will work to repair this rupture by sharing with the service user their understanding of the difficulties within the relationship, as understood through problematic patterns highlighted on the map, and how together they may go about stepping out of these patterns. In addition, when working together for a number of weeks, the ending of sessions can feel difficult; therefore the therapist will prompt discussion about the ending at different points throughout the therapeutic contract, to keep it on the agenda and give space to think about the difficult feelings coming to an end may elicit.

As we progress through the course of this book, you will notice how frequently we talk about the therapist/service user relationship. Never underestimate its significance or value in understanding what difficulties are occurring for the service user, as no doubt they will be re-enacted within the therapeutic space.

Karen says:

> *I think you have to be able to click with the therapist as well. If it's someone you can't like jog along with each week, it's not going to work, is it? I liked her firmness. You know I liked the way she'd put me straight if I was like going too deep into something or seeing something that wasn't there. She'd bring me back, and I liked that about her, I like thinking along those thoughts, you know let's take it back, it's getting you back on track, isn't it?*

Andrew says:

> *You know I've left some therapies and you almost feel like you are best friends with the therapist. With her I didn't. I didn't feel lost, so there wasn't that rejection at the end because I didn't fail. It was absolutely fantastic because I could go somewhere, and I could tell somebody anything and not be judged by them and not worry them because again I think it is entirely what was needed, and I didn't want her to react.*
>
> *There is nothing that isn't on the table. I will tell you everything you know, my deepest, darkest, horriblest thoughts if you wanna hear them I'll tell you them and that has allowed me to be a lot more open since.*

The structure of CAT

You will often hear CAT being spoken about as a 'short-term' and 'time-limited' approach to therapy. As mentioned earlier, Ryle originally developed CAT as a brief approach to manage the increasing waiting list and pressure for therapy within his service. An early discussion that the therapist has with the service user (usually once assessment is complete) is the 'contract' to CAT sessions. Within this conversation, together they collaboratively agree on the number of sessions which will take place, depending upon need; in CAT this is generally 8, 12, 16 or 24 sessions. The benefit of the contract to CAT is twofold, not only because it ensures equitable access, but it also allows for the ending to be considered from the start, with the final session being acknowledged all the way through the process. The value of this is to be able to reflect together on any fears the service user may have about therapy coming to an end, how they may manage without the therapy, and to manage the attachment within the therapeutic relationship. It is also about being transparent and holding both the therapist and service user to account in terms of the potential pull to avoid discussing the ending, Therefore, once the total number of sessions has been agreed, it is imperative that, in all but exceptional circumstances, this number of sessions is adhered to. Extending the contract midway through therapy may serve to increase the potential separation anxiety and decrease the service user's perceived sense of ability to manage outside of sessions.

For the purpose of this section, we are going to consider the structure of a typical 16-session contract of CAT in more detail, as this is the most frequently used number of sessions which is, whilst an arbitrary number, a reasonable amount to start off on a journey of change. Contracting to CAT usually takes place following an initial assessment session to gather details about the service user's needs. Succeeding sessions are then counted as part of the contract (e.g., sessions 1–16). Whilst each of these aspects will be addressed in more detail throughout the book, we will touch upon them briefly here.

Assessment (sessions 1–3)

For CAT, the initial assessment is usually an extended one, with the therapist gathering information about the service user's life history within the initial three sessions. Here, the therapist delves deeper into understanding the significant life events for the service user, important relationships and a narrative of their life story. Alongside this, the therapist will ask the service user to take home the *psychotherapy file* to complete (usually at the end of session 1 or 2), as a means of reflecting upon their own patterns and difficulties outside of sessions (see Chapter 6 for further information). Upon returning the psychotherapy file, the therapist and service user will consider together the information that has been gathered and think about how this relates to life experiences and the shared understanding they have begun to construct. Early mapping may begin, with the therapist tentatively suggesting key features of the service user's story and such features then being written down in the beginnings of a state map (which will be described in detail later).

Reformulation letter (session 4, sometimes 5 or 6!)

The aim of assessment is for the therapist to glean enough information to allow them to begin to write the *reformulation letter* outside of sessions, in preparation for sharing in session 4. This is the recommended time in which Ryle suggested the reformulation letter be shared, as a means of beginning to develop the shared understanding of the service user's reciprocal roles and problematic procedures, in the context of key relationships and experiences they have had from childhood through to the present day.

In reality, we recognise that sharing the letter at session 4 is not always possible. At times, the therapist may not fully feel prepared to write the letter; they may not feel as though the assessment is adequately completed or that they have not had time to discuss it in clinical supervision (particularly important for all CAT practitioners in training or those new to the approach). In these instances, with discussion and agreement with the service user, this letter may come at session 5 or, at a push, session 6.

The reformulation letter will be created by the therapist in a form which is best understood by the service user – usually this is in written form – and two copies are taken to the session. The therapist reads the letter aloud to the service user whilst the service user follows with their own copy. This approach is particularly valuable for the service user to encounter both a visual and verbal presentation of the letter, in the hope this increases their familiarity with the contents. Upon having shared the letter, the therapist will offer space to await the service user's response, following which, the letter will be used together to begin to support the mapping and aim-directed middle phase of therapy.

Middle phase (sessions 5 or 6 - 15)

The subsequent sessions, post reformulation letter, are the ones classed as the 'middle phase' in CAT and are often the sessions that form somewhat of an enigma in the literature. This is possibly due to the variety of ways in which therapists work throughout these sessions or the abundance of models that can be drawn upon due to the integrative nature of its approach. Despite this, however, there are central key features to the middle phase of CAT that therapists tend to follow.

Firstly, the recognition of the target problem, and thus the goal-orientated aims for therapy, direct the focus for change. For example, a service user who recognises their target problem as being "I find it hard to take care of myself" may agree to work with the therapist on a target problem procedure (TPP) of feeling not good enough, which results in them avoiding their own personal needs and thus neglecting their own self-care. From here, the therapist will help the service user begin to *recognise* a TPP by increasing their observing eye both within and outside of sessions, through noticing when patterns are occurring. The constant presence of the CAT map within the room in therapy will aid the therapist in discussing patterns as they notice them occur within their shared dialogue, and thus pointing them out on the map.

It is hoped that as the service user's observing eye begins to develop, they become more skilled at recognising patterns, which will then lead to a shift in being able to step out of the maintaining difficulties and to find suitable exits. Exits are considered part of the *revision* phase in therapy, which leads the service user to notice how they can do things differently and will hopefully have a beneficial effect on their lives. To return to the earlier example of the service user who found it hard to take care of themselves, they may find therapy helps them to begin to notice times in which they do not feel good enough and to begin to trial thought challenging, alongside actively implementing self-care strategies. In doing so, the service user may then begin to feel a sense of belonging, thus stepping out of the neglecting-to-neglected, self-to-self reciprocal role. The therapist will promote the monitoring of exits on the CAT map, allowing the service user to visibly see areas of change.

The middle phase of CAT always keeps the ending as a central feature, with the therapist 'counting down' the number of completed sessions at the start of each session (e.g., "today we are at session 7 out of 16"). As the therapy reaches significant milestones, such as the midpoint and latter few sessions, the therapist speaks in more detail about the approaching ending and what this feels like for the service user. This will allow for any difficulties and fears to be verbalised, and credit given to the uncertainty that endings bring, alongside how the service user will continue to maintain progress outside of therapy.

Ending (session 16)

Within the final session (or sometimes the penultimate session), the therapist will share a *goodbye letter* with the service user. Once again, this letter is written outside of the sessions in preparation for session 16. The letter comprises the therapist's reflections on the progress the service user has made, the exits they have discovered, any difficulties that have occurred throughout the therapy, as well as challenges they may continue to face into the future. The aim of the goodbye letter is to provide the service user with a transitional object that they can take outside of sessions to reflect upon their development, as well as to integrate both the 'good and bad' parts of therapy – for example, the improvements the service user has made, alongside the pain that an ending can bring.

In addition to the therapist sharing a goodbye letter, the therapist will have offered the service user the opportunity to write a goodbye letter outside of therapy and to bring it to the final session. The service user has complete choice in whether or not they write a letter; they will be asked, however, to reflect upon what they have achieved within therapy, what has been difficult and where the therapy leaves them now (either through the letter or verbally within the final session).

Three-month review

At session 16, the therapist will discuss with the service user the structure of CAT in offering a three-month review appointment. This session is intended as a one-off appointment to review the service user's progress post-therapy, and not as an extension to the therapeutic contract. The three-month review appointment will be planned at the end of session 16 and will comprise discussions surrounding how the service user has managed post-therapy, any additional progress they have made and any further difficulties they have encountered. It allows the therapist to signpost the service user back to the use of the therapeutic tools developed throughout the CAT contract and to consider how they will continue to progress following the three-month review.

Conclusion

In this chapter we have briefly considered the origin of CAT, focusing both upon the social circumstances and need that shaped its time-limited approach and on Ryle's drive for theoretical integration and a common language for the psychotherapies. We have considered the relative contribution of the C in CAT – including the active, collaborative, goal-directed structure and the focus on interlocking patterns of problematic thoughts and behaviours that it shares with cognitive therapies such as CBT. The key analytic concepts (the A in CAT) have been explored with particular focus upon the ideas of transference and projection of different sorts. The key phases, or three Rs of CAT – namely, reformulation, recognition and revision – have been explored, with particular reference to what we might think of as the fourth, all important R – the therapeutic relationship. Lastly, we have described what might be thought of as a 'typical' 16 session CAT structure. We hope that this will give the beginning CAT therapist an outline before we consider each of the elements of CAT in further detail in the forthcoming chapters.

References

Association for Cognitive Analytic Therapy. (2016). Dr Tony Ryle, 1927-2016. *Reformulation*. https://www.acat.me.uk/page/tonys+biography

Beck, A. T. (1967). *Depression: Clinical, Experimental and Theoretical Aspects*. Harper & Row.

Denman, C. (2001). Cognitive-Analytic Therapy. *Advances in Psychiatric Treatment*, 7, 243–256. https://doi.org/10.1192/apt.7.4.243

Fairburn, W. R. D. (1954). *An Object-Relations Theory of the Personality*. Basic Books.

Freud, S. (1911/1958). Psycho-analytic notes on an autobiographical account of a case of paranoia (dementia paranoides). In *The Standard Edition of the Complete Works of Sigmund Freud* (Vol.12, pp.1–82). Hogarth Press.

Freud, S. (1912/1958). The dynamics of transference. In *The Standard Edition of the Complete Psychological Works of Sigmund Freud* (Vol.12, pp.97–108). Hogarth Press.

Kelly, G. A. (1955). *The Psychology of Personal Constructs. Volume 1: A Theory of Personality*. Norton.

Knobloch-Fedders, L. (2008). The importance of the relationship with the therapist. *Clinical Science Insights: Knowledge Families Count On*, 1, 1–4.

Maloney, R. (2008). Reformulation: Education, collaboration, or coercion? *Counselling Directory*.

Ogden, T. (1982). *Projective Identification and Psychotherapeutic Technique*. Jason Aronson.

Rayner, K., Thompson, A. R., & Walsh, S. (2011). Clients' experience of the process of change in Cognitive Analytic Therapy. *Psychology and Psychotherapy: Theory, Research and Practice*, 84, 299–313. https://doi.org/10.1348/147608310X531164

Ryle, A. (1991). *Cognitive-Analytic Therapy: Active Participation in Change. A New Integration in Brief Psychotherapy*. Wiley.

Ryle, A. & Kerr, I. (2002). *Introducing Cognitive Analytic Therapy. Principles and Practice of a Relational Approach to Mental Health.* Wiley.

Ryle, A. & Kerr, I. (2020). *Introducing Cognitive Analytic Therapy. Principles and Practice of a Relational Approach to Mental Health.* Wiley.

Ryle, A., Kellett, S., Hepple, J. et al. (2014). Cognitive Analytic Therapy at 30. *Advances in Psychiatric Treatment,* 20(4), 258–268. ISSN 1355-5146. https://doi.org/10.1192/apt.bp.113.011817

Tanner, C. (2002). Target problems: The Focus in a CAT Therapy. *Reformulation,* Summer, p. x.

Vygotsky, L. S. (1978). *Mind in Society: The Development of Higher Psychological Processes.* Harvard University Press.

Winnicott, D. W. (1965). *The Maturational Processes and the Facilitating Environment.* International Universities Press.

Young, J. E. (1990). *Cognitive Therapy for Personality Disorders: A Schema Focused Approach.* Professional Resource Exchange.

4 Who is Cognitive Analytic Therapy for?

Introduction

Before we begin to look at the 'how-to' of CAT, we need to consider in more detail who CAT is appropriate for. There are a number of different ways in which we can look at this, from a generational perspective (e.g., across the lifespan), to a service perspective (e.g., learning disabilities, health, forensics), to a cultural perspective. Whilst the evidence base for CAT is often critiqued as being limited, we will look at the current literature available in each of these areas, whilst holding in mind the consideration of *practice-based* evidence and how you will see that CAT is often used in numerous services within the NHS because of its relational approach.

It is also helpful to think about potential difficulties that service users often present with, and how these can be considered when determining whether CAT is appropriate, alongside the contraindications to using CAT, for example, when it may do more harm than good. In a nutshell, it is important to consider 'why' we choose CAT as an approach, alongside 'when' it can be most beneficial (e.g., in terms of service user readiness). Karen and Andrew help us consider when they felt CAT was most appropriate for them within the course of their life experiences.

CAT across the lifespan

As mental health services are generally structured across the lifespan (child and adolescent mental health services, adult mental health services, and older adult mental health services), it is important to stop for a moment and consider ageing in relation to the use of CAT. As Ryle (ACAT, 2016) founded CAT at Guy's and St. Thomas' Hospital (based within a busy inner-London setting), over the course of ten years of him working at the base, he assessed around 1 per cent of the adult population within the catchment area, for CAT. CAT lends itself to a 1:1 therapeutic approach given its relational focus, and emphasis on collaborative working. Therefore, it is no surprise that the majority of the limited evidence base has focussed on working in adult populations. In a systematic review in 2014, albeit now relatively old, Calvert and

DOI: 10.4324/9781003308256-4

Kellet looked at the evidence base for using CAT. Out of 25 of the final studies, 23 recruited from an adult population and suggested the effectiveness of using CAT for a range of presentations from acquired brain injury to eating disorders to survivors of childhood sexual abuse. The review reported limited findings for the effectiveness of CAT in dissociative disorders. More generally, much of the adult evidence base for CAT is suggestive of using CAT in the standardised way, which will be discussed further within this book. CAT literature in other settings across the lifespan (e.g., child and older adult) focusses more so on the adaptations which can be made to the approach, in order to increase its accessibility to the younger and older populations.

Varela (2016) spoke of the uses of a CAT-informed approach with young children. Here, attention is paid to engaging collaboratively with the child and parent, to offer adaptations such as co-creation, creativity, joint activity between parent and child, and the therapeutic partnership, allowing for all involved to be curious participants of the therapy. Adapting the approach to be child-centred, Varela (2016) suggested a play-based assessment, altering language to meet the needs of the child (e.g., suggesting a problem circle instead of a sequential diagrammatic formulation), having collaborative sessions alongside 1:1 sessions with either the parent or child, and using metaphors, toys and analogies to explain the problem and find suitable exits. Whilst the evidence base for working with children is limited, such adaptations have been well received. Ougrin et al. (2008) considered such adaptations when working with young people presenting with self-harm. They consider the use of a therapeutic assessment utilising a CAT approach in comparison to assessment as usual. The therapeutic assessment differed to assessment as usual, as it included developing a map, identifying a target problem, developing motivation to change, considering potential exits, and providing a summary in an understanding letter. Ougrin et al. (2008) found that young people assessed using this approach were more likely to engage with community follow-up than their matched-assessment-as-usual peers.

More attention in the literature has been paid to the use of CAT with older people. In particular, Hepple and Sutton (2004) provide a thought-provoking and emotional consideration of using CAT with older people in their well-respected book *Cognitive Analytic Therapy and Later Life: A New Old Age Perspective.* 'Within the book they reflect on how working with older people can be both the 'same' and 'different', as it is not necessarily age that affords adaptation, but the experiences that come with later life. In particular, existential issues such as What will happen when I die? How do I live without my loved one? and 'What is the meaning of life?' become fundamental challenges in older age and at times can require person-to-person empathic dialogues, to work through them. Age is a construct which is experienced by individuals in different ways – for example, being chronologically old versus being physically old versus being psychologically and socially old. When an older adult experiences a dilemma in any one of these areas (e.g. "I need a hip replacement, but I still want to garden as I have done in the past" or "Modern technology is beyond me now yet I need to go online to make a doctor's appointment"), emotional turmoil can be heightened. Often there can be more than one of these challenges being faced at a time, particularly with individuals experiencing multiple losses (e.g., of loved ones, their role through retirement, cognition, capability, driving; Sutton & Gaskell, 2016).

Sutton and Gaskell (2016) highlight how emotional neglect can often be re-experienced by older people within services, as their needs are left unmet. When considering cohort and generational effects within older people's mental health services, it is important to recognise the social and political experiences this generation may have lived through. As the current older generation grew up in the 1930s and 1940s, they may have experienced a whole host of challenges due to the war and illness. For example, this could include evacuation from parents and the family, subsequent adaptation to impersonal situations, being of large families where parents struggled to put food on the table or loss of parents (either permanent or temporary), to name a few (Sutton & Gaskell, 2016). Children within this era may have encountered emotional neglect due to these issues, or the 'keep a stiff upper lip' belief, or where parents were cold or harsh to their youngsters. Within older age, such experience of emotional need may be heightened once again, as the requirement to be cared for is re-experienced. Sutton and Gaskell (2016) highlight the importance of offering a 'meeting eye' within services, whereby staff are trained to reduce shame and stigma and to attend to the service users' emotional needs.

Within older people's services, CAT has been found to be beneficial not only for service users, but also for their carers. Hamill and Mahony (2011) worked with carers of individuals with dementia, to attend to their wellbeing, emotional needs and experience of living grief, encountered through the role. The CAT approach adopted was found to provide a non-threatening, therapeutic space to make sense of patterns the carers were experiencing, to find new possibilities within the caring role and to understand endings and the grieving processes in relation to dementia.

The above considerations of CAT across the lifespan are not exhaustive by any means but do highlight the usefulness of using CAT within these settings, through adapting its approach and being creative, to meet the needs of the service user.

CAT in differing settings

Alongside the use of CAT across the lifespan, the approach has been readily utilised in a number of other clinical settings (e.g., learning disability, health and forensics), some of which have been noted within the literature for the last 25 years (Fosbury et al., 1997; Pollock & Belshaw, 1998). The overarching consensus within the literature when working in each of these settings on a 1:1 basis with service users is the importance of CAT in stepping back from the 'diagnosis' and focussing on the relationship to the self and others. In addition, the use of contextual reformulation (using CAT as a formulatory approach working with staff teams) is also highlighted as valuable in helping staff to understand the reciprocal roles (RRs) and procedures that they may inevitably become caught up within, in relation to the service user (Jenaway, 2011; Marshall et al., 2014; Moss, 2007).

In regard to working with individuals with a learning disability, as early as 1992, Sinason challenged the notion that people with a learning disability do not benefit from psychotherapy. She identified the presence of both cognitive and emotional intelligence, and that whilst cognitive intelligence may be affected, emotional intelligence for such service users does remain intact. Through adaptation of the CAT model (through language, diagrams and pictures), Crowley (2002) acknowledged that individuals with a learning disability can both utilise and understand the model effectively. Lloyd and Clayton (2013) within their book entitled *Cognitive Analytic Therapy for People with Intellectual Difficulties and Their Carers* provide examples of adapted CAT tools for working with this population. Moss (2007) acknowledged that the use of CAT and its development in working within a learning disability setting has been largely down to the CAT practitioner's creativity in using the model flexibly.

Psaila and Crowley (2006) noted that four main RRs can be found when working with individuals with a learning disability, particularly due to their seeming to have fewer RRs to draw upon, leading to greater distress at times. Such RRs identified are abusing/bully to abused/victim; damaging to damaged; rejecting to rejected and abandoning to abandoned. Idealised RRs often found in this population are rescuing/caring to rescued/cared for and special/perfect to learning disabled. As staff members working within this area, one's own attitudes (or collective attitudes of a team) may lead to such RRs being reinforced. Contextual reformulation in teams (which is also touched upon later in this chapter) can therefore allow for exploration of the relationship with the service user, and to find ways in which such patterns are not reinforced within interventions.

The use of CAT in forensic services has broadly taken a similar journey, through adapting CAT when working 1:1 and considering the use of CAT more systemically within teams. Pollock, Stowell-Smith and Göpfert in their 2006 book entitled *Cognitive Analytic Therapy for Offenders: A New Approach to Forensic Psychotherapy* recognise how CAT has been applied with promise to a number of different presentations and thus its use within forensic services is also hopeful. They approach the book with expertise from a service-user presentation perspective, considering the adaptability of CAT to a number of different groups such as the treatment of child sex offenders, to parents within prisons, to stalking offenders, to community perpetrators of domestic violence. Once again, the requirement to be creative and innovative within therapy due to the restricted reciprocal role repertoire forensic service users may have (Mitzman, 2010) is well considered in the literature. Pollock and Belshaw (1998) discuss, using case examples, the adaptations required for service users who are offenders, such as: using engaging and applicable language (to consider how the offender understands their own relationship with the victim); developing jointly constructed sequential patterns (with an aim to understand the motivations for the offence) and to adapt interventions to meet the service user's needs (often in this population through behavioural management techniques).

Marshall et al. (2014) pioneered the initial considerations of developing reflective settings for staff members working within forensic and secure services. Moon (2015) acknowledged how staff teams often face the challenge of offering security and therapeutic space for service users in forensic settings whilst also managing aggressive and violent outbursts. Through the use of CAT as a relational model, training and routine reformulation sessions within the team can allow for a common language for staff to understand their interactions with service users. Having management onboard to offer this more indirect approach to working is essential, as contextual reformulation can provide scaffolding to the team, allowing staff to support one another in order to achieve the team's true potential (Moon, 2015). In their book *Reflective Practice in Forensic Settings: A Cognitive Analytic Approach to Shared Thinking*, Marshall and Kirkland (2021) consider in-depth the use of an integrative and reflective approach to working with forensic service users on an individual level, as well as service and organisational approaches to thinking relationally and reflecting on practice.

With regards to the use of CAT in healthcare settings, clinical outcomes have emerged for health difficulties including medically unexplained symptoms (Jenaway, 2011), obesity (Hill, 2015) and diabetes (Fosbury et al., 1997). The first considerations of the use of CAT within health care settings was that of Fosbury et al. (1997), who completed a trial of the therapy with individuals with poorly controlled type 1 diabetes. Where service users were randomly allocated to a trial of 16-session CAT or 14–16 sessions of diabetes nurse specialist education (DNSE), results indicated the longer term benefit of CAT with both glycaemic control and interpersonal difficulties showing improvement both immediately and at a nine-month follow up; this was in comparison to the DNSE group who showed improvement in glycaemic control following sessions but no longer-term effects on this or within interpersonal difficulties.

Considering the use of a psychological approach in healthcare settings can be difficult, particularly as the service user may be invested in a medical treatment approach to 'cure' the illness, rather than considering any psychological involvement or consequences of the health condition. This can be particularly the case in services treating chronic pain and medically unexplained symptoms. The value of the CAT approach, however, is to be able to consider the service user's relationship with the diagnosis, rather than suggesting that a psychological condition is the 'cause' of the illness. Jenaway (2011) explains this further in her work in a service for medically unexplained symptoms (MUPS). She identifies that those who are wedded to the idea that their pain is due to a physical cause can be most difficult to engage. CAT, however, allows for exploration that the 'cause' of the pain is not important, more so how the service user relates to the pain and how this then triggers specific coping strategies (which are likely to be linked to past experiences of illness). She uses the analogy that even with a broken leg (which has a clear physical cause), we will still react to it psychologically (e.g., pushing oneself too hard before it has healed or feeling low in mood because one's independence has been removed).

Within chronic pain, Davis (2017) speaks to the challenge that such service users' experience when recognising that the pain is 'never ending'. Service users with chronic pain are often faced with medical procedures (e.g. injections, medication, operations) that can leave them to feel 'done to', whereas CAT allows space to 'be with' the service users, considering who or what the pain represents to them relationally, how to attend to the meaning of pain through integrating the body and the mind, and how to grieve the loss of 'what could have been' had the pain not existed. In a preliminary evaluation of the use of CAT for adults with chronic pain, Baronian and Leggett (2020) found significant effects on self-efficacy, wellbeing and psychological distress, post-therapy, for service users who had completed eight sessions of 1:1 CAT.

Such findings of the use of CAT more broadly within specialist settings are encouraging, and additional research is needed in order to further develop the evidence base. The generation of literature from a practice-based evidence perspective is suggestive of how useful CAT is in daily practice, and how adaptable and creative the approach can be to meet the needs of each individual clinical population.

CAT and cultural considerations

Like many Westernised models of psychological therapy, CAT was developed by a white male who occupied a position of relative privilege and power in comparison to many who may work within and seek the support of mental health services. The theories and models that CAT draws from were similarly developed largely by white men and women from the Westernised world. Additionally, whilst we cannot assume that people from ethnically minoritised backgrounds are not accessing CAT or being represented within CAT research, the lack of demographic information on the culture and ethnicity of participants within the published CAT research to date, coupled with what we know about the barriers to accessing health services for those from minoritised groups, is enough to cause concern.

Whilst we need to hold in mind the potential cultural biases inherent in the model, it would of course be equally as discriminatory to assume its inapplicability to individuals from non-Westernised or ethnically minoritised backgrounds (in CAT terms, perhaps this would be a dilemma between *either* being blind to the influence of culture on the one hand *or* diminishing that which may be of value, on the other). CAT theory and tools were developed within a Westernised context, but unlike many other models of psychological distress, CAT makes explicit its consideration of 'the values and structures of the wider culture' (Ryle & Kerr, 2002, p. 2) in developing and maintaining the sense of self.

The creativity of the relationally based mapping process within CAT prompts us not just to consider the intra- and interpersonal, but also to consider the interaction between the individual and all levels of the 'ecological systems' (Bronfenbrenner, 1979) that surround them. This may include their relationship with culture, ethnicity, geographic location, gender, sexuality, socioeconomic status, religion, and the changing sociohistorical circumstances across their lifespan.

So, how might the individual practitioner ensure that cultural considerations are a key part of their practice? Treisman (2021) defines cultural humility as "the ability to maintain an interpersonal stance that is other-oriented (or open to the other) in relation to the aspects of cultural identity that are most important to the person". This hints at the importance of recognising how the multiple identities (visible, invisible, voiced and unvoiced) that someone has may intersect – seeing people as unique individuals within a wider context rather than as part of a "homogenous group". She goes on to explain that cultural humility involves an "active engagement and a lifelong ongoing process of self-reflection and self-critique whereby the individual not only learns about another's culture, but starts with an examination of their own beliefs, biases, assumptions, values and cultural identities" (Kumagai & Lypson, 2009; Tervalon & Murray-Garcia, 1998).

Cultural humility and responsiveness are clearly values and behaviours fostered by the individual therapist in relation to the individual service user, rather than being inherent to any particular model of therapy. However, several CAT clinicians and authors have made important contributions in considering how CAT may intersect with themes of culture, diversity and power. For example, Brown and Msebele (2011) present a CAT understanding of the reciprocal roles involved in racism and argue that the concepts of race and racism should be acknowledged within the therapy room in order to pave the way for a more authentic and respectful dialogue.

This points to both the ongoing work we must do ourselves as individual therapists as well as the relational stance that it is crucial we adopt if we aim to be responsive to diversity in our work with others. Like Treisman, we would strongly emphasise the position that cultural humility is not a 'deficit model' – whilst we must take care not to avoid or silence areas of concern – this must be balanced with a drive to celebrate and respect difference, honouring strength, survival and resources. For an introduction to this topic, or to support the reader in this continuing journey, we would recommend Treisman's chapter titled "Cultural Humility and Responsiveness" (Treisman, 2021, pp. 309–349).

CAT and diagnoses

As we have no doubt mentioned elsewhere, one of the features of the CAT model is that it can be applied trans-diagnostically. Unlike CBT, there are no 'diagnosis specific' conceptualisations within CAT, although of course, certain early experiences or ways of surviving may tend to go hand in hand with particular patterns of roles and procedures. The important thing, though, is that reformulations and sequential diagrammatic reformulations (SDRs) are constructed organically and individually, 'from the ground up', with the service user. Reciprocal roles and traps/dilemmas/snags do form a template of sorts, but the content of these and the ways in which they are linked are unique to each service user. This makes it possible to develop conceptualisations that are completely bespoke to the individual. 'Symptoms' may well appear on maps but tend to be seen as a consequence of underlying problematic patterns (themselves created from the need for survival strategies), rather than as the direct target of intervention themselves. Whilst a discussion on the validity and usefulness of psychiatric diagnosis is not within the scope of this text, the interested reader is referred to *The Power Threat Meaning Framework* (Johnstone et al., 2018) for a full exploration of the social and relational contexts of emotional distress as an alternative to diagnosis.

Despite this, we recognise that the world in which CAT operates is still largely diagnosis-led – statutory mental health services speak the language of diagnosis and often subscribe to a medical model understanding of psychological distress. There is also often the need for research investigating the efficacy of psychological therapies to recruit participant groups who all meet the criteria for the same diagnosis; this is (for the most part) also reflected in the organisation of the National Institute for Health and Care Excellence guidelines. For these reasons if no other, it is perhaps important to ensure that there can be a dialogue between the CAT model and the concept of diagnostic categories.

Whilst we would argue that CAT can be a good 'first offer' for service users with a variety of presenting difficulties, it is worth consulting the evidence base to consider what the first-line recommendation for treatment is when difficulties appear to cluster around a particular diagnostic category. Whilst it is important to be transparent with the service user in terms of what the evidence base suggests, it is equally important to consider service user choice. For example, CBT may be the treatment of choice for many specific anxiety-based disorders such as obsessive compulsive disorder, generalised anxiety disorder, post-traumatic stress disorder and panic. However, CAT may be indicated where CBT has been previously tried but has been unsuccessful or had limited success, where there are comorbidities or key relational difficulties, or where there is a strong service user preference for working relationally.

Although CAT has traditionally been linked to work with more 'complex' presentations, the model is also showing promise as a treatment for anxiety and/or depression in people re-presenting in a number of different settings: for example, in primary care talking therapies settings (Owen et al., 2023), in group CAT within primary care (Martin et al., 2021) and in demonstrating comparable outcomes to CBT for people with anxiety and depression in the context of complex relational problems, within the 'high intensity' tier of Improving Access to Psychological Therapy (IAPT) services (Wakefield et al., 2021). As referred to above, previous research has suggested the acceptability and utility of the model for people with more 'complex' presentations such as people with psychosis (Taylor et al., 2015, 2019), people with a diagnosis of personality disorder (Chanen et al., 2008; Clarke et al., 2013) and female survivors of childhood sexual abuse (Calvert et al., 2015).

Andrew says:

> *There is a feeling that comes with depression and when you are at your lowest and it's a bloody terrifying place to be and I think for CAT to work you need to be not in that feeling but close enough so you can still know what you felt like. I can't remember what it felt like to be at my worst, but up until recently I could still put myself back in that position and remember those feelings of utter hopelessness and that I'm not in control of my life and it's like heading to a wall at 90 mph and you know the crash is coming but there's nothing you can do about it. It's like sheer terror. And I think I needed to be far enough away from that for CAT to be able to actually happen but close enough to remember it, so it is critical when it happens.*

CAT and its contraindications

Unlike other models, CAT has no expectations with regards to the degree of 'psychological mindedness' needed as a prerequisite to engagement, nor are there any 'suitability scales' which will tell you how well matched the model is to your service user's traits and abilities. Indeed, the main aim of the therapy may be to develop this level of self-awareness and reflexivity. Despite this (and as with all therapies), there does need to be a readiness and willingness to explore one's own internal world and a motivation to engage with the work and make changes. However, as Ryle and Kerr (2002) point out, the early sessions of CAT are often motivating in themselves as they create the conditions under which a greater degree of self-reflection can begin to develop. Whilst people who are severely depressed or actively psychotic/experiencing a current manic episode may not be readily accessible to a psychological therapy without other interventions taking place first/alongside this, both of us have successfully continued to work with existing service users who have experienced episodes of severe low mood or mania during active CAT. The same is likely to be true for cases which involve high levels of risk to self or others – a thorough risk assessment is paramount and multi-disciplinary or even multi-agency collaboration and care may become necessary; however, the decision as to what level of risk can be acceptably worked with ultimately rests with the individual therapist.

As will be discussed in more detail in Chapters 5 and 7, the importance of informed consent to therapy within the context of trauma-informed care cannot be overstated. Many people who come for therapy will have experienced relationally based trauma at some point – CAT explicitly explores the stories and historical narratives of our lives; the decision to tell these stories must rest with the service user, however. In this sense, whilst there are probably very few outright contraindications to an offer of CAT, a collaborative consideration of the relative risks of harm versus benefits must be made together with the service user to ensure that the timing of therapy is right for them.

Karen says:

> *I think CAT had to come at a time when I had my feelings under control and also it wasn't going to trigger [them] either. I was like confident in myself that I could open up about everything and not like, you know that will get me manic, having feelings kick in. So for me I think it had to come at that right time and it was at that time it was safe for me you know because I did get emotional about my past but I knew it wasn't going to make me poorly, so I had to try and address things and get through, you know I couldn't have a conversation about my childhood without crying and like reliving things, but I thought no I've got to strip it right back and talk to someone who can help me make sense of everything. And that's exactly what I did. Years ago, I wouldn't have been able to.*

Andrew says:

> *I don't think it could have been any earlier, you know looking back the fire-fighting had to happen, you know to sit in a burning building and talk about stuff, you know you need not to be on fire. So, because you're in that fight or flight, there's too much panic going on, you know so as much as I said this was my last chance, I would slide back, but I would never slide back to the bottom.*

CAT and its different uses

Across all services, lifespan and specialist settings, CAT can also be used indirectly. Whilst the focus of this book is to attend to the direct practice of CAT with service users, we also want to acknowledge the vast application that CAT can have outside of this.

CAT has been shown to be effective in many other ways, such as:

- Being used as a contextual reformulatory approach (e.g., with staff members to aid understanding of a service user's presentation when the CAT practitioner is not directly involved in the service user's care; Moss, 2007);
- Five-session CAT consultancy (to work for a short period of time with the service user and care co-ordinator to formulate and guide an intervention plan; Carradice, 2013);
- Staff training and reflection (particularly in forensic services to aid staff reflection in challenging situations; Marshall & Kirkland, 2021);
- Organisationally in staff teams (when team dynamics are difficult or sickness rates are high; Craven-Staines & Finch, 2024); and
- For staff wellbeing (e.g., employee support, taking care of staff's mental wellbeing; Craven-Staines, 2019).

Using CAT as a contextual reformulatory approach is one which has been shown useful across a number of services. Returning to a learning disability setting as an example, Moss (2007) highlighted that there may be certain maladaptive patterns that staff members can become drawn into when working with service users. Having reflective space within teams to reformulate and understand the patterns is a key method in allowing staff not to inhabit such roles and patterns or to reciprocate them. Within learning disability settings, Lloyd and Williams (2004) identified common RRs that staff can be drawn into, such as: persecuting-to-persecuted; ideally caring-to-ideally cared for; rejecting-to-rejected; punishing-to-punished and controlling-to-compliant. When such roles occur, teams can become 'split' as staff members occupy the opposing end of the role in relation to the service user. Such splitting can in turn lead to stress and burnout in staff groups (Moss, 2007). Working at a staff level to develop contextual reformulations can pre-empt such breakdowns within the support system.

Whilst these are just a few of the ways in which CAT can be used creatively outside of the therapy room, it is important for the developing practitioner to be aware of their existence, in order to explore further CAT's application in differing ways, as they become more skilled and confident in utilising CAT as an approach.

Conclusion

It is hoped that this chapter helps the reader explore the clinical utility of CAT above and beyond more formal, structured 1:1 sessions. CAT has been explored and effectively embedded widely in a number of service settings, across the lifespan and with a number of differing presentations. It is important for the CAT practitioner to be aware of the cultural limitations of CAT and to truly, relationally explore the meaning of wider equality and diversity experiences for the service user. As the CAT practitioner feels more skilled within their underpinning knowledge of the theory and its use in practice on a 1:1 basis, applying CAT's systemic and organisational approaches can also be great additions to service settings.

References

Association for Cognitive Analytic Therapy. (2016). Dr Tony Ryle, 1927-2016. *Reformulation*. https://www.acat.me.uk/page/tonys+biography

Baronian, R. & Leggett, S. J. (2020). Brief cognitive analytic therapy for adults with chronic pain: A preliminary evaluation of treatment outcome. *British Journal of Pain*, 14(1), 57–67. https://doi.org/10.1177/2049463719858119

Bronfenbrenner, U. (1979). *The Ecology of Human Development*. Harvard University Press.

Brown, H. & Msebele, N. (2011). Black and White Thinking: Using CAT to think about Race in the Therapeutic Space. *Reformulation*, Winter, pp. 58–62.

Calvert, R. & Kellet, S. (2014). CAT a review of the outcome evidence base for treatment. *Psychology and Psychotherapy*, 87(3), 253–277.

Calvert, R., Kellett, S., & Hagan, T. (2015). Group Cognitive Analytic Therapy for female survivors of childhood sexual abuse. *British Journal of Clinical Psychology*, 54(4), 391–413. https://doi.org/10.1111/bjc.12085. Epub 2015 May 28. PMID: 26017051.

Carradice, A. (2013). 'Five Session CAT' Consultancy: Using CAT to guide care planning with people diagnosed within community mental health teams: Brief summary report. *Reformulation*, Winter, pp. 15–19.

Chanen, A. M., Jackson, H. J., McCutcheon, L. K., Jovev, M., Dudgeon, P., Yuen, H. P., Germano, D., Nistico, H., McDougall, E., Weinstein, C., Clarkson, V., & McGorry, P. D. (2008). Early intervention for adolescents with borderline personality disorder using cognitive analytic therapy: Randomised controlled trial. *The British Journal of Psychiatry: The Journal of Mental Science*, 193(6), 477–484. https://doi.org/10.1192/bjp.bp.107.048934

Clarke, S., Thomas, P., & James, K. (2013). Cognitive Analytic Therapy for personality disorder: Randomised control trial. *British Journal of Psychiatry*, 202, 129–134. https://doi.org/10.1192/bjp.bp.112.108670

Craven-Staines, S. (2019). Reflecting on the role of Cognitive Analytic Therapy in the provision of care for mental health staff in an Employee Psychology Service. *International Journal of CAT & RMH*, 3, 94–106.

Craven-Staines, S. & Finch, J. (2024). CAT consultancy for enhancing team functioning. In L. Brummer, M. Cavieres, & R. Tan (Eds.), *Oxford Handbook of Cognitive Analytic Therapy*. Oxford University Press.

Crowley, V. (personal communication). In Ryle, A. & Kerr, I.B. (2002). *Introducing Cognitive Analytic Therapy: Principles and Practice*. Wiley, 173.

Davis, M. L. (2017). "Never-ending hurt": How CAT can help inform the management of chronic pain. *Reformulation*, Summer, 16–21.

Fosbury, J. A., Bosley, C. M., Ryle, A., Sönksen, P. H., & Judd, S. L. (1997). A trial of cognitive analytic therapy in poorly controlled type I patients. *Diabetes Care*, 20(6), 959–964. https://doi.org/10.2337/diacare.20.6.959

Hamill, M. & Mahony, K. (2011). 'The long goodbye': Cognitive Analytic Therapy with carers of people with dementia. *British Journal of Psychotherapy*, 27, 292–304. https://doi.org/10.1111/j.1752-0118.2011.01243.x

Hepple, J. & Sutton, L. (2004). *Cognitive Analytic Therapy and Later Life: A New Perspective on Old Age*. Routledge.

Hill, L. (2015). CAT and obesity: My reflections. *Reformulation*, Winter, 8–9.

Jenaway, A. (2011). Using Cognitive Analytic Therapy for medically unexplained symptoms: Some theory and initial outcomes. *Reformulation*, Winter 2011, 53–55.

Johnstone, L., Boyle, M., Cromby, J., Dillon, J., Harper, D., Kinderman, P., Longden, E., Pilgrim, D., & Read, J. (2018). *The Power Threat Meaning Framework: Towards the Identification of Patterns in Emotional Distress, Unusual Experiences and Troubled or Troubling Behaviour, as an Alternative to Functional Psychiatric Diagnosis*. British Psychological Society.

Kumagai, A. K. & Lypson, M. L. (2009). Beyond cultural competence: Critical consciousness, social justice, and multicultural education. *Academic Medicine: Journal of the Association of American Medical Colleges*, 84(6), 782–787. https://doi.org/10.1097/ACM.0b013e3181a42398

Lloyd, J. & Clayton, P. (2013). *Cognitive Analytic Therapy for People with Intellectual Difficulties and Their Carers*. Jessica Kingsley Publishers.

Lloyd, J. & Williams, B. (2004). Exploring the use of cognitive analytic therapy within services for people with learning disabilities and challenging behaviour. *Clinical Psychology and People with Learning Disabilities*, 2(3), 20–22.

Marshall, J. & Kirkland, S. (2021). *Reflective Practice in Forensic Settings: A Cognitive Analytic Approach to Developing Shared Thinking*. Pavillion Publishing and Media Ltd.

Marshall, J., Freshwater, K., & Potter, S. (2014). Using Cognitive Analytic Therapy within a forensic setting: An overarching relational model. *Forensic Update*, 115. https://doi.org/10.53841/bpsfu.2014.1.115.46

Martin, E., Byrne, G., Connon, G. & Power, L. (2021). An exploration of group cognitive analytic therapy for anxiety and depression. *Psychology and Psychotherapy: Theory, Research and Practice*, 94 (s1), 79–95. https://doi.org/10.1111/papt.12299

Mitzman, S. F. (2010). Cognitive Analytic Therapy and the role of brief assessment and contextual reformulation: The jigsaw puzzle of offending. *Reformulation*, Summer, 26–30.

Moon, L. (2015). My experience of Cognitive Analytic Therapy (CAT) within a secure forensic setting. *Reformulation*, Winter, 12–15.

Moss, A. (2007). The application of CAT to working with people with learning disabilities. *Reformulation*, Summer, 20–27.

Ougrin, D., Ng, A. & Low, J. (2008). Therapeutic assessment based on Cognitive-Analytic Therapy for young people presenting with self-harm: Pilot study. *Psychiatric Bulletin*, 32(11), 423–426. https://doi.org/10.1192/pb.bp.107.018473

Owen, K., Laphan, A., Gee, B. et al. (2023). Evaluating Cognitive Analytic Therapy within a primary care psychological therapy service. *British Journal of Clinical Psychology*, 00, 1–11. https://doi.org/10.1111/bjc.12430

Pollock, P. & Belshaw, T. (1998). Cognitive analytic therapy for offenders, *The Journal of Forensic Psychiatry*, 9(3), 629–642, https://doi.org/10.1080/09585189808405378

Pollock, P.H., Stowell-Smith, M., & Göpfert, M. (Eds.). (2006). *Cognitive Analytic Therapy for Offenders: A New Approach to Forensic Psychotherapy* (1st Ed). Routledge. https://doi.org/10.4324/9780203929537

Psaila, C. L. & Crowley, V. (2006). Cognitive Analytic Therapy in people with learning disabilities: An investigation into the common reciprocal roles found within this client group. *Reformulation*, Winter, 5–11.

Ryle, A. & Kerr, I. (2002). *Introducing Cognitive Analytic Therapy. Principles and Practice of a Relational Approach to Mental Health*. Wiley.

Sinason, V. (1992). *Mental Handicap and the Human Condition: New Approaches from the Tavistock*. Free Association Books.

Sutton, L. & Gaskell, A. (2016). Meeting with older people as CAT practitioners: Attending to neglect. *Reformulation*, 6–13.

Taylor, P. J., Hutton, P., & Wood, L. (2015). Are people at risk of psychosis also at risk of suicide and self-harm? A systematic review and meta-analysis. *Psychological Medicine*, 45(5), 911–926. https://doi.org/10.1017/S0033291714002074

Taylor, P.J., Perry, A., Hutton, P., et al. (2019). Cognitive Analytic Therapy for psychosis: A case series. *Psychology and Psychotherapy: Theory, Research and Practice*, 92, 359–378. https://doi.org/10.1111/papt.12183

Tervalon, M. & Murray-Garcia, J. (1998). Cultural humility versus cultural competence: A critical distinction in defining physician training outcomes in multicultural education. *Journal of Healthcare for the Poor and Undeserved*, 9(2), 117.

Treisman, K. (2021). *A Treasure Box for Creating Trauma-Informed Organizations: A Ready-to-Use Resource for Trauma, Adversity, and Culturally Informed, Infused and Responsive Systems*. Jessica Kingsley Publishers.

Varela, J. (2016). "Playing" with CAT - Using a CAT informed approach with young children and their families. *Reformulation*, Summer, 6–10.

Wakefield, S., Kellett, S., Simmonds-Buckley, M. et al. (2021). Improving Access to Psychological Therapies (IAPT) in the United Kingdom: A systematic review and meta-analysis of 10-years of practice-based evidence. *British Journal of Clinical Psychology*, 60, 1–37. https://doi.org/10.1111/bjc.12259

5   Setting the scene

Introduction

Having set the scene in terms of the overall structure, application and key components of CAT, we now move into the 'how-to' chapters of the book. Often, when starting out in CAT, sessions can feel daunting to the practitioner, particularly in being able to articulate the approach clearly to the service user. It can feel overwhelming to consider how much or how little to share when describing the concept of CAT and what sessions may look like. This tends to come more naturally with time and practice, and CAT practitioners often develop their own unique ways of explaining the model. This chapter aims to provide you with an example of how to set the scene in therapy whilst considering issues relating to choice, power and informed consent within the initial sessions. It is important to bear in mind that every CAT practitioner will have their own style and way of discussing CAT with the service user; therefore, what we present here are suggestions of techniques that you can use as a developing therapist, and over time you will develop your own approach which will feel comfortable for you. Finding your own unique way of describing concepts is often helpful, as it will feel more natural to you and the service user, who will not experience it as a rehearsed script.

On reflecting on her initial session, Karen says:

> *So obviously when I was introduced to her [therapist] then she told me what it was gonna be about, you know, and then how we were gonna look at things that had happened in the past to change my, to kind of like to change your thought process now and acceptance of what's happened. Yeah, it was all a bit confusing really when I look back; I didn't really understand.*

DOI: 10.4324/9781003308256-5

Andrew recalls what things were like for him prior to attending his first CAT session:

> *As for me it was similar; I didn't know what it was, nothing was explained to me it was just, it was the first time that I had done something proactively and when I sought help before it had been through either the crisis team or Mind [a mental health charity] and that was kind of firefighting when it was just a case of that, this was the first time that kind of looked at everything. I spoke to the doctor first and had my meds upped and like I said I didn't know what to expect but at that time I was I was melodramatic shall we say in that if this doesn't work then that's it, I'm gone you know because I can't live like this anymore.*

These quotes perhaps highlight that in the gap between being referred for CAT and attending the initial session, service users may know very little about the model or what to expect. The first session of therapy can be an incredibly emotive and confusing time (as Karen and Andrew describe), and so whilst it feels important to do a 'good enough' job of explaining what CAT is, what it looks like and what it will try to help with, we perhaps also need to hold in mind that when emotions are running high, it will be difficult to take in too much complex information. Therefore, we aim to simplify the description of CAT as much as possible.

Before we begin to explore how you might set the scene and explain something about CAT to your service users, though, we'd like to ensure you have an initial grasp of the key terms that are used in CAT so that you can move from a position of 'jargon' into a place where you feel comfortable in explaining some of these complex terms to others. The role of the CAT practitioner is to 'bridge the gap' between the theoretical literature and the model in practice, so that the theory can be used in an accessible way. The following section will guide you through easy-to-understand definitions of the key terms, and if relevant, which aspect of the psychological theory the concept relates to. They are not intended to be an exhaustive list that should be memorised, but more so a guide to simplify understanding.

What is a target problem?

A target problem can be defined as the main issue to be worked upon in therapy. It is different to a 'presenting problem' in that whilst the therapist and service user may identify some of the key presenting difficulties or symptoms together, the target problem describes the difficulties *relationally*, often through recognising what the service user is struggling to do, in relation to themselves or others. Tanner (2002) described a target problem as being the main problem which feels difficult enough to drive the person to seek help or find a way of making it better. Imagine a service user presenting to you in therapy with low mood, withdrawing from day-to-day activities, and experiencing self-deprecating thoughts. Throughout assessment, you consider together some of the main reasons as to why the service user is experiencing such difficulties. The service user speaks of times throughout childhood when they encountered feelings of embarrassment, judgement and humiliation in front of others, both at school and at home. More recently, at work, they were left to feel shamed and self-conscious when reprimanded by a boss in front of colleagues. Here, jointly identified target problems could be 'I struggle to speak my mind' or 'I find it difficult to be around others'. These target problems then allow key goals to be developed to work on in therapy (e.g., in this case to aim to find ways of being assertive or to develop skills and confidence in social situations).

What is a target problem procedure?

Target problems usually occur due to the repetitive pattern(s) underpinning them; these are often termed the Target Problem Procedure(s) (TPP; Catalyse, 2013). A TPP shows how the target problem is maintained due to a sequence of belief, aim, plan, action, response and feedback (which can be remembered by the mnemonic BAPARF). So, thinking back to the case above; feeling ashamed, humiliated and self-conscious in relation to the experience at work, the service user:

- Thinks 'I am useless, and no one will ever like me' (*belief*)
- Wishes that they could feel in control again *(aim)*
- Decides to step back from being around others, as this always causes them problems *(plan)*
- Puts the plan into practice through withdrawing from work and social events *(action)*
- Feels low in mood and lacking in energy *(response)*
- Continues to feel useless due to not having spoken their mind, and having dropped out of social situations *(feedback)*

In a contract to CAT, the therapist and service user identify one or two target problems which are underpinned by around four or five TPPs (also known as problematic procedures, or 'patterns' when named in therapy). TPPs are often broken down into three main types of patterns that people find difficult to change. Such TPPs are spoken about in detail by Ryle and Kerr (2020), and examples are highlighted in the psychotherapy file. These TPPs are:

> **Traps** – *circular patterns of thoughts and behaviour*, where a belief often leads to an action, which in turn resultantly leads to the belief being confirmed. This can be considered as a 'vicious circle', where the person becomes stuck and is unable to find a helpful way out of the pattern.

Dilemmas – this pattern is usually depicted by an *either/or* option where the person feels forced to choose between two polarised choices. Either decision they make will create an unpleasant consequence for the individual, leading to the difficulty being maintained.

Snags – in these patterns, individuals often *stop an appropriate goal before it is started*, due to believing that their achievement is not deserved or allowed. The self-fulfilling prophecy in sociological terms is an example of this (e.g., the idea that a false belief influences what a person does, which in turn then shapes reality; Merton, 1948).

What is a reciprocal role?

Reciprocal roles (or sometimes 'roles' for ease of use in therapy) are the developed sense of self we form throughout childhood in relation to another (usually the parent or other central caregiver). We experience emotional reactions to the other person's behaviours or dialogue, which we internalise (adopt or take on as our own). From this experience, we then learn how to engage in similar interactions with others. So, for example: if I experience my mother as punishing of my behaviour, I feel upset, punished and guilty. I learn it feels bad to do things wrong and learn to take on the role of 'punishing' also. Reciprocal roles are often drawn to depict two parts of a relationship (e.g., a reciprocal, or give-take interaction; see Figure 5.1). Jenaway (2019a) coined the term 'relationship roles' reporting that 'reciprocal roles' make them sound more complicated than they actually are.

As a result of internalising such interactions, the person can then learn how to enact the role in relation to themselves and other people. A helpful way to explain the self in relation to others and self to self is highlighted in Figure 5.2.

In life, we all have a mixture of both healthy and more problematic reciprocal roles. An example of a healthy reciprocal role is 'caring-to-cared-for', where

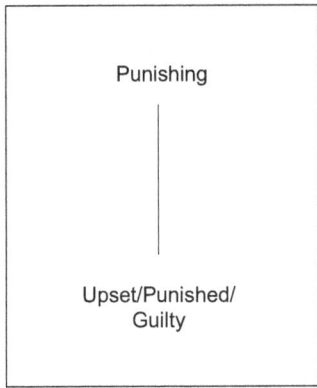

Figure 5.1 An example of a reciprocal role.

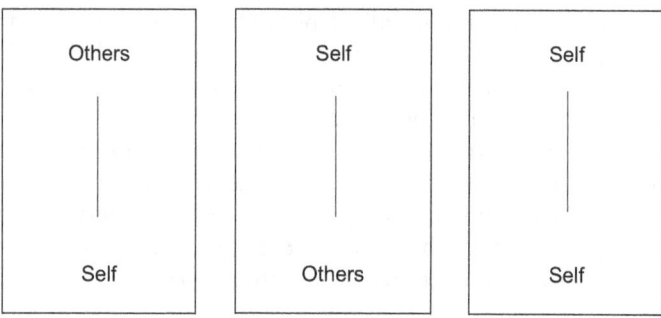

Figure 5.2 The reciprocity of relationships.

a person experiences what it is like to be cared for, and thus learns how to care for others and themselves. An example to bring this to life could be the way a very young child might play at looking after their teddy or dolly, feeding them and comforting them in the same way their own parent has with them. This neatly demonstrates the way that relational interactions are experienced, internalised and then repeated with others. We can have a large range of reciprocal roles to draw upon, having learnt from a variety of experiences we have encountered within our life.

However, for some, as a result of experiencing persistently harsh, abusive or painful relationships with others, the repertoire of roles can become narrowed, and we often fall into similar situations over and over again, making it difficult to find a way out. Such repeated patterns are often re-enactments of past relationships in current relationships. In CAT, we refer to this as 'joining the dance'; we find others that are similar (or with interlocking/reciprocal patterns) to us, who can be pulled (or moved) into complementary ways of being and relating. We form an intricate pattern of relating that repeats the 'to and fro' of difficult interactions. It can often feel like 'groundhog day' within our relationships, where reciprocal role interactions are repeated, for example: a child who has experienced domestic violence within their upbringing may find themselves in a romantic relationship with a controlling or violent other. These interactions are better known in CAT terminology as *Reciprocal Role Procedures*, patterns of interrelating that can be enacted in different ways: others do it to me, I do it to myself or I do it to others, or I draw others in so it feels like they are doing it to me (Potter, 2010).

Often CAT practitioners in training can find it tricky to map out the reciprocal roles clearly. In order to help with this, it is useful to think of the top end of problematic roles as the *pain-inducing* end (e.g., the behaviour/thought/dialogue that creates pain within the self or other). This top end of the role can often be thought of as the 'doing to' position, and thus often ends with an 'ing' (e.g., criticis*ing*, controll*ing*, abus*ing*). On the opposite end, the bottom part of the problematic role is often known as the *pain-experiencing* end (e.g., the core pain, or intense emotional reaction as a result of the interaction). This can be depicted as 'done to', being written as an 'ed' (e.g., criticis*ed*, controll*ed*, abus*ed*). It is important to remember that within reciprocal roles, for a person to be in the pain-inducing end, they must too have suffered the pain-experiencing end, in order to have internalised the emotion. For example: if I am on the experiencing end of a critical mother, I can feel criticised, hurt and upset. As a result, however, I then learn to be critical of myself and others. My mother, too, however, must have experienced the pain experiencing end of the 'criticising-to-criticised' role within her own life. CAT aims to clearly step away from a victim- or parent-blaming position. Patterns can be characteristics within all of us, as a result of our basic human instincts to relate to one another and the self.

What is a state map?

When beginning to consider areas of an individual's life that they are struggling with, a CAT practitioner usually considers strong emotions the person has and particular *states of mind* that they experience. These states of mind often comprise emotions, memories, behaviours and thoughts that all relate to certain roles we are involved in (Catalyse, 2013). Through development within our childhood, we can develop higher-level, cognitive strategies ('meta-procedures') that allow us to integrate and move between states relatively seamlessly.

For individuals who have experienced a neglecting, punitive or abusive upbringing, the ability to integrate such states of mind can be impacted, and thus the shift between 'self states' can appear unexpected, disjointed or abrupt. These ways of thinking have often been employed as a way of surviving such difficult experiences. Through beginning to name states in the early stages of therapy, and mapping them onto paper, the therapist is helping the service user notice such swift shifts in feelings, with an aim to find a position of integration. The state map often underpins the development of the sequential diagrammatic reformulation (SDR), as it emphasises the key areas of difficulty the service user is struggling with and can then be used within the session through understanding the states together and beginning to employ the theoretical aspect of CAT within mapping. For example, if the state map identifies a state of being withdrawn, exhausted and pulling away from others, the CAT practitioner may discuss with the service user what leads them to this state as a means of beginning to map out a problematic procedure. The service user may indicate times in which they feel their needs are not met by others, which often leads them to feeling low in mood and pulling away from interaction. In terms of mapping, a neglecting-to-neglected reciprocal role may be identified, leading to a *trap* of feeling low in mood, that 'no one wants me; I'm no use to anyone' therefore 'I'm better off on my own', and then withdraw from interactions, being left to feel neglected once again (see Figure 5.3 for state and mapping example).

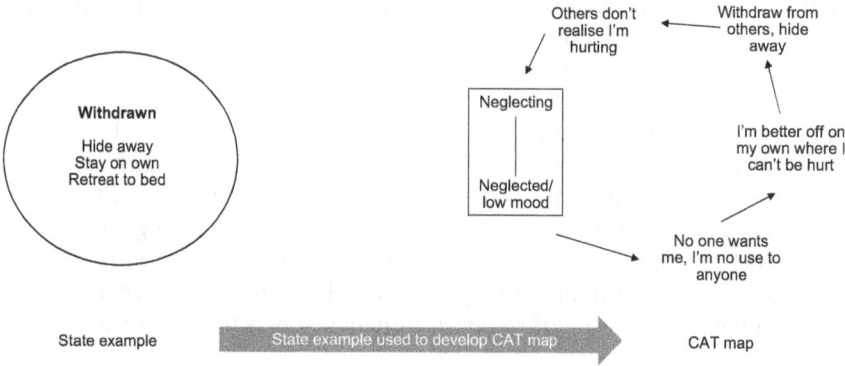

Figure 5.3 State and CAT mapping.

What is a Sequential Diagrammatic Reformulation (SDR)?

The SDR is often referred to more simply as a 'CAT map' in therapy. This is the mode of understanding the service user's difficulties from a visual perspective and brings together the use of reciprocal roles and problematic procedures. Ryle (1998) explained that the SDR 'sets out to describe the core reciprocal role repertoire'. It is here that the integration of theories is clearly seen, from the cognitive behavioural aspects of the TPPs to the analytic components of the reciprocal roles.

What is the observing eye?

When explaining the CAT approach, practitioners often find it useful to highlight the importance of reflection within therapy, as a means of beginning to notice problematic patterns as they occur. When developing a map with the service user, the practitioner may draw an eye (often on a top corner of the map) to depict the process of standing back from our usual, automatic ways of being to becoming aware of our own roles and patterns by observing ourselves more closely (Jenaway, 2019b). Generally, the recognition that the therapist may have an 'observing eye' on the problematic patterns also can be helpful. The scope throughout therapy is then to support the service user in developing their own observing eye.

What is core pain?

The term 'core pain' is one frequently used in CAT to refer to the central issue, especially in relation to the unknown and unmanageable feelings, which are hoped to be discovered and understood through therapy (Boa, 1998). It is the place on the map that is ultimately the most painful one for the service user to occupy. Core pain can be depicted on the map in colour or pictorially to highlight its significance (e.g., red and jagged for hurt and anger). In 1998, Ryle stressed the danger of the term 'core pain' due to its suggestion that the therapist should rescue the service user from the emotion or ignore any potential projection. Core pain can be a multitude of emotions that the service user experiences. Metaphorically, it can be considered as the centre of an onion, which can be the most difficult place to get to as there are layers to peel first. Core pain can be considered as within the centre of an individual, deep inside; however, it can be the most unpleasant, excruciating feeling when experienced (sometimes named the 'dreaded place'). Due to the intense emotion, the individual will try to escape this, through engaging in survival strategies which can later become problematic patterns, no doubt resulting in the repetition of the same or another reciprocal role. If the core pain is felt within sessions, the their can support the service user in staying with the emotion, rather than trying to avoid it, through finding alternate ways out of the problematic patterns.

What is a healthy map?

When introducing CAT to the service user, it can often feel emotionally 'heavy', particularly as the focus is on the difficulties that the service user is experiencing and currently feeling stuck with. Focus on the positives and healthy ways of relating can also be beneficial for the service user, through noticing their strengths and helpful coping strategies. As the service user continues to find alternate, new ways of coping throughout therapy, these too can be added to the healthy map, through identifying healthy reciprocal roles and procedures.

What are exits?

It is often helpful to name with the service user early on in the discussion of the therapeutic approach that the ultimate aim of therapy is to find ways of stepping out of the TPPs into alternate, more helpful ways of being. These are termed 'exits' in CAT and are usually mapped onto the SDR. One way of doing this is through creating a numerical key, linking the place on the map where the service user stepped out of the TPP to what they did that was different.

Below we describe a potential way to explain RRs:

In CAT we often talk about this idea of 'reciprocal roles'. You don't need to worry about what they are called, but the key idea is that, based on the ways that parents and key others have related to us as we were growing up, we all internalise these 'roles' – which are like our templates or blueprints of how we expect others to relate to us and how we behave towards others.

   For example (starts to draw out a 'loving-loved' reciprocal role on a piece of blank paper), if a parent behaves in a loving way towards us, we will learn what it feels like to be loved. But we don't just learn what it feels like to receive love, by virtue of having experienced this; we also learn how to love others and how to love ourselves. A good example of this is when you see a small child taking care of and cuddling their dolly; they are re-enacting that caring, loving way of relating, that they have been on the receiving end of from a parent, towards their doll. This would be an example of what we might think of as a healthy reciprocal role.

We can all also have less-helpful reciprocal roles; a common example of this, which lots of us might be able to relate to is criticising-to-criticised (draws out reciprocal role on paper). If we have been criticised by a parent whilst we were growing up, we learn what it's like to be on the receiving end of criticism, but we also learn how to be critical towards ourselves and maybe even towards others. Of course, it's painful to feel criticised, so we understandably want to get away from this bottom half of the role. To get away from this place, we might do things like trying to be perfect all the time to please others, in the hope that then they won't criticise us (draws out arrow moving away from bottom of reciprocal role). However, as we know, it's not possible to please everyone all of the time, and perfection is a myth – when we inevitably can't keep this up, we are open to being criticised all over again (if not by others, then by ourselves!). So, the basic idea with reciprocal roles is that they might start off as being other-to-self, but that they can also then become self-to-self and self-to-other. We typically refer to this top part of an unhelpful role as the 'pain-inducing end' and this bottom half as the 'pain-experiencing end'. It's also important to remember that it's our experience that counts, it doesn't mean that our parent was intentionally trying to be critical towards us, but if that's how we experienced it, then that's what matters.

Choice, power and informed consent

Whilst we set the scene for therapy, we will no doubt also be focussing on other considerations. The acknowledgement and exploration of issues surrounding power are crucial in all psychological therapies, not just CAT. A substantial proportion of the general population, and an even larger number of those experiencing mental health difficulties, will have experienced interpersonal trauma at some point in their lives. The experience of trauma is almost universally entwined with the idea of power, and more specifically, power differentials. In this context one of the relational aims of CAT *must* therefore be to acknowledge the power imbalance that exists between therapist and service user and to work on minimising this as far as is possible. This involves a recognition of the further harm (and indeed re-traumatisation) that can be caused in therapy when power imbalances are not attended to and are acted out or perpetuated. CAT is perhaps in a uniquely accessible position in terms of understanding, naming and stepping back from these imbalances. In line with the principles of trauma-informed approaches, we will now consider the importance of choice and consent in CAT. It should be noted that whilst we are focussing here on the importance of addressing these issues early on in the process of contracting to CAT, they continue to be equally as important in all other stages of therapy.

Whatever the 'source' of a referral for psychological therapy, it is crucial to establish 'where' the difficulty lies and who will benefit the most from the potential changes to be made. As experienced therapists, we have both been asked to assess people for therapy in situations where it quickly becomes clear that the person themself is not the driving force behind the request. Often, their presenting patterns of relating, thinking, feeling and behaving are not so much a problem for themselves as they are for the people close to them. The pressure from external sources to embark upon the work of therapy can sometimes be immense (and not without good reason); this presents us, as therapists, however, with an ethical and practical dilemma which cannot be ignored. This, of course, is not unique to working within the CAT model, but we would argue that CAT is particularly well placed to explore and work through these conflicts.

Whilst many professional codes of conduct refer to the importance of gaining informed consent (e.g., HCPC Standards of Proficiency: Practitioner Psychologists, 2023; NMC The Code, 2018), there is often a dearth of exploration of what this might mean in practice, and interestingly, ACAT's own Code of Ethics and Practice (2018) does not explicitly explore the idea of *consent to treatment*. We might of course assume that this is implicit when a service user seeks treatment, however, as discussed above, this is not necessarily the case. So, as well as an explanation of what CAT is and what it aims to do, what else might someone need to know to give genuine informed consent to engaging in CAT?

We propose here some key considerations for the beginning therapist with regards to choice, power and informed consent in CAT. This is by no means an exhaustive list nor an in-depth exploration of the ethical principles underpinning these points; we do hope, however, that these considerations will provide a useful scaffold in thinking and talking about consent.

1. *Informed consent as an ongoing, bidirectional process* – consent to treatment, and in fact, consent to assessment for treatment, should be discussed with potential service users at the earliest possible opportunity. This should not be seen as a single conversation that, once done, can be "ticked off" and put to one side for the remainder of the work. In fact, it may be important to revisit this conversation at different stages of the therapy. We know that the first session can be a confusing and emotive one and as such, some of these conversations may benefit from repetition or re-exploration at different points. Ultimately, the service user needs to have sufficient information about the therapy and its potential risks and benefits to be able to make an informed decision about consent to treatment; the points below therefore expand upon the areas which may be helpful to discuss to facilitate this process.

2. *Confidentiality and its exemptions* – a full awareness of the limits to confidentiality should be the cornerstone of seeking informed consent to all talking therapies. It can feel tempting to 'brush over' this issue for fear of evoking difficult feelings or questions for the service user, perhaps also for fear of limiting a therapeutic relationship before it has even truly begun. However, a trusting therapeutic relationship will be based on honesty and transparency, and as such it is crucial to inform service users under which circumstances confidentiality may need to be breached (usually if there is a significant risk to self or others or any safeguarding concerns), how this will be approached and, more generally, the safeguards in place to maintain the confidentiality of their information.

3. *The basics in terms of duration of sessions, length of treatment* – as therapists in training we are usually well socialised to what therapy 'looks like' – however, this may not be so for those with whom we work. Some basic information about the length and frequency of sessions, the venue (and crucially, what choices there are regarding this) and the likely duration of treatment can be useful in helping service users decide if this is something they feel ready and able to embark upon (see boundaries and contracting sections later in the chapter for more information).

4. *The techniques that will be used in therapy* – all therapists (even within the same model) work slightly differently, and it is therefore useful for potential service users to know a little about how you work before they consent to treatment. As we have already outlined in this chapter, this might include a broad overview of the approach as well as more specific information, in lay terms, about the techniques that will be used within therapy. It can be helpful to provide the service user with some brief written material on this or to direct them to material on the internet so that they can read and digest this in their own time, outside of sessions.

5. *The range of other psychotherapies which are available* – whilst it is important not to overwhelm the potential service user with information, it is also crucial to be honest and transparent about the other therapeutic approaches which may be suitable for them. This will particularly be the case if they prefer a certain way of working, or where there is a robust, established evidence base for certain approaches in relation to their presenting difficulties.

6. *The evidence base and 'common factors'* – as stated above, it is important to refer to what we know about the evidence base for therapies in different circumstances; there is an important caveat here, however. It is not uncommon for research to be based upon populations which are not particularly representative of who we see in the consulting room. A critical appraisal of other potential limitations of the evidence base for psychological therapies is outside the scope of this text; however, what does seem to be demonstrated time and again is the importance of what are known as 'common factors' in determining therapeutic outcome, regardless of the model being used (e.g., Wampold, 2015).

7. *Potential harms, risks and benefits* – again, there may be a pull to skim over information about risks and potential harms when attempting to engage someone in a therapeutic intervention; transparency and honesty here, however, will only serve in the development of a trusting therapeutic relationship. It is certainly important to be aware that embarking upon any psychological therapy is an emotionally challenging process and that things will be stirred up and may feel worse before they get better. This can, of course, be presented alongside the typical benefits that others who've experienced CAT typically report.

Whilst we would encourage beginning CAT therapists to consider each of the issues above in setting the scene for therapy, there will be many ways to do this sensitively within the early sessions. For example (depending on the service you work within), it may be that such material is provided in written format to be read in between sessions and brought back for discussion. Depending on how the service user is feeling and what they need within the early sessions, it may not be possible to consider all of these issues straightaway, and in fact it may be counterproductive to even attempt this in some cases. For example, it may feel important to discuss consent and confidentiality as early as possible; it may be that considerations around what the treatment would look like and what the alternatives are can wait until later on in the process of assessment for therapy.

Boundaries and contracting

Boundaries within psychological therapies provide the frame within which difficult emotions can be held and attended to whilst also ensuring feelings of safety are maintained for service user and therapist. The layers of boundary include the moral and legal frameworks which guide our practice, as well as the more subtle emotional and relational boundaries which must be attended to (Finlay, 2015). A consistent, reliable and predictable frame is of course a relational intervention in itself and can contribute significantly to healing when the service user's boundaries have been breached in the past. Different therapists, working within distinct modalities across diverse settings will naturally adhere to slightly different boundaries. A psychoanalytic therapist, for example, may discourage contact from service users outside of formal sessions. In other therapeutic modalities however, such as Dialectical Behaviour Therapy, service users are *expected* to contact their therapist in between sessions in certain circumstances. Whilst all schools of therapeutic practice and ethics are clear that therapists should not overstep the boundary from a professional into a personal relationship with service users, and would encourage us to think carefully about the management of 'dual relationships', individuals differ on the flexibility of their boundaries with regards to other elements of the therapeutic relationship. How flexible are you around the considered use of self-disclosure as a therapeutic tool, for example? Are you able to offer sessions outside or whilst walking in nature if the clinic room is too triggering or trapping for the individual that you are working with? Will you accept phone calls from your service user in between planned sessions? Rather than applying rigid boundaries carte blanche, we would encourage you to carefully consider what you feel comfortable with as a therapist, to ask yourself what is in the service user's best interests, and always to make use of supervision in discussing boundaries and the decision to flex these. It's always easier to set out our boundaries from the start of therapy, so that service users know what to expect and can ask questions about these upfront.

When contracting to CAT, the therapist and service user need to be open and honest about the boundaries surrounding the therapy, in order to manage expectations and to develop a safe environment. In general, sessions occur on a weekly basis, preferably on the same day, same time each week (to maintain a 'therapeutic frame', Knox & Cooper, 2015). In these conversations, it is best to agree with the service user the number of sessions that will take place and plan the dates together from session 1 right through to the final session. In doing so, it can be made clear with the service user when breaks will occur and what will happen if sessions are cancelled or not attended. For example, some practitioners will make a boundary around not replacing non-attended sessions in all but the most unavoidable or extreme of circumstances, whereas cancelled sessions may be replaced. Such planning can also help with the 'countdown of session numbers' at the start of each appointment, where the therapist names with the service user the session number, in order to keep the ending in sight. In addition, having an awareness of when breaks in therapy will occur can be comforting for the service user, so that they can be discussed in prior sessions, and the service user is mindful of them approaching. Each session will usually last 50 or 60 minutes in duration; the length of sessions will also be contracted to with the service user. Ensuring this discussion occurs is important so the therapist can prompt the service user when the session is nearing an end and make sure they do not over run.

It can also be helpful to discuss the structure of CAT, highlighting when the service user should expect the reformulation letter, what will take place in the 'middle sessions' (e.g., homework and monitoring), and when the goodbye letter will be shared. In addition, it is useful at this point to advise that a review appointment will be offered post-therapy, to check in on the service user's progress.

Karen and Andrew speak of the emotional demands of the therapeutic encounters and the way in which they experienced CAT across the course of their contracts.

Karen says:

I think there's weeks where you don't really feel like going and we take a lot to it, and you take a lot away from it. A lot of tears shed, well for me there was, and you can feel absolutely drained from it. But you know that, you get things to work on yourself and then you know, when you go back as each week goes on, you see changes.

Andrew says:

And like I said the emotional toll it took on you, you know the day I had therapy, yeah, I did nothing else. Would probably go home and sleep or just you know you're almost [in] a vegetative-like state and you know there were days when I'd come back and I'd think I'm not going back next week I can't do that again but like, like we've said, you don't remember absolutely all of it, but you live your life by it, and it's still affecting me now.

Conclusion

It is hoped that through this chapter you have begun to become acquainted with the main terminology used in CAT, and how these concepts relate to the therapeutic approach itself. The terms 'reciprocal roles' and 'target problem procedures' (traps, dilemmas and snags) form the underpinnings of both the reformulation letter and the sequential diagrammatic reformulation (SDR, also known as a CAT map). The importance of considering power, choice and informed consent within the therapeutic contract is highlighted, alongside the need to agree to a contract of therapy together, and the value of boundaries. It is hoped that this chapter provides the developing CAT practitioner with an understanding of the considerations they need to make before engaging with a service user, alongside deliberation of how to begin to have discussions with the service user about what CAT entails. Each of these issues is the starting point of engaging with the service user, and important to hold in mind when embarking on the assessment and throughout the therapeutic contract.

References

ACAT. (2018). Code of ethics & practice. https://www.acat.me.uk/page/code+of+ethics+and+practice

Boa, C. (1998). SDR's for beginners. *Reformulation*, ACAT News, Autumn.

Catalyse. (2013). *Glossary of CAT terms and concepts.* https://catalyse.uk.com/training/glossary-of-cat-terms-and-concepts/

Finlay, L. (2015). Holding, containing and boundarying. In L. Finlay (Ed.), *Relational Integrative Psychotherapy.* https://doi.org/10.1002/9781119141518.ch5

Health and Care Professions Council. (2023). *Standards of Proficiency: Practitioner Psychologists.* HCPC.

Jenaway, A. (2019a). Relationship roles - All about CAT. http://acat.org.uk/

Jenaway, A. (2019b). The "Observing Eye" in CAT - All about CAT. http://acat.org.uk/

Knox, R. & Cooper, M. (2015). *The Therapeutic Relationship in Counselling and Psychotherapy.* Sage.

Merton, R. K. (1948). The self-fulfilling prophecy. *The Antioch Review*, 8(2), 193–210. https://doi.org/10.2307/4609267

Nursing and Midwifery Council. (2018). *The Code: Professional Standards of Practice and Behaviour for Nurses*, Midwives and Nursing Associates, NMC.

Potter, S. (2010). Words with arrows: The benefits of mapping whilst talking. *Reformulation*, Summer, 37–45.

Ryle, A. (1998). Sequential diagrams. Reflections and suggested revisions. *Reformulation*, Autumn.

Ryle, A. & Kerr, I. (2020). *Introducing Cognitive Analytic Therapy. Principles and Practice of a Relational Approach to Mental Health.* Wiley.

Tanner, C. (2002). Target problems: The focus in a CAT therapy. *Reformulation*, Summer.

Wampold, B. E. (2015). How important are the common factors in psychotherapy? An update. *World Psychiatry*, 14, 270–277.

6 Cognitive Analytic Therapy assessment tools

Introduction

Prior to thinking about how we formally conduct a CAT assessment, we find it helpful to consider the appropriate objective measures and CAT tools that can be useful aids in gathering additional information from the service user. This chapter aims to introduce you to two of the main objective measures used in CAT, which can be beneficial in measuring pre- and post-therapy outcomes. These are the Inventory of Interpersonal Problems, also known as the IIP, and the Personality Structure Questionnaire (PSQ). The main CAT tool which informs the assessment is known as the psychotherapy file, and this chapter will consider its development, content and variety of different types. Chapter 7 will then determine how to introduce and utilise the psychotherapy file within the assessment session.

Objective measures

It is always pertinent to measure outcomes for the service user, often for service requirements, but also for reference at the end of sessions to reflect on progress. Objective measures are beneficial for not only determining change, however. They can also be useful for the therapist to gather more information about the service user's current presentation within the assessment. For CAT in particular, understanding the service user's ability to relate interpersonally, as well as their capacity to integrate different parts of the self is important, and such measures can support this process.

The Inventory of Interpersonal Problems

In 1979, Horowitz identified three dimensions within interpersonal relating through the scaling of statements made by service users within their own psychotherapy. These three dimensions included: the degree of involvement the service user feels in relation to others (e.g., intrusiveness vs avoidance); how intentional their involvement with others is (e.g., dominance vs submissive); and finally, the nature of their involvement with others (e.g., friendly

DOI: 10.4324/9781003308256-6

vs hostile). Such dimensions were the underpinning theory to the Inventory of Interpersonal Problems, which was later developed by Horowitz et al. in 1988. The original IIP is a 127-item measure which taps into a number of different types of interpersonal problems and aims to help service users and the therapist determine sources of interpersonal distress. In order to respond to each item, the service user reports how much difficulty or distress they feel in relation to the item, on a scale of 0–4 (with 4 being a greater level of distress). Within the measure, the first 78 items begin with 'it's hard for me to …' and the remaining 49 items begin 'this I do too much …'.

Horowitz et al. (1988) studied the psychometric properties and clinical application of the IIP through 103 service users completing the measure both at the start and end of their time on a waiting list for brief psychotherapy. On both occasions, the factor analyses identified the same six subscales, indicating high test-retest reliability and internal consistency. The study was, however, critiqued by Barkham et al. (1996) due to its limited sample size and having a sample within which the sex was too highly skewed towards females. In addition, the measure was critiqued for eliciting responses that were either too high or too low.

Whilst there was agreement that the measure taps into several types of interpersonal problems, there was disagreement in how many distinct dimensions are represented. Alden et al. (1990) constructed a circumplex scale for IIP, on the understanding that interpersonal problems can be organised on two dimensions, split into eight sectors (or octants). From this, a secondary version of the IIP was developed named the Inventory of Interpersonal Problems-Circumplex (IIP-C), which is a 64-item questionnaire divided into eight scales. Upon evaluation, the IIP-C was noted to have strong psychometric properties, which remained when translated into 12 different languages.

As the research into the measure continued, establishing a more accessible version for use within practice was needed. Barkham et al. (1996) developed a shorter version, namely, the Inventory of Interpersonal Problems-32. The 32 items are equally distributed across the eight subscales, with items continuing to consider 'things I find too hard' (e.g., to join in groups) or 'do too much' (e.g., get irritated). The five-point scale of 0 (not at all) to 4 (extremely) was maintained. Exploratory analysis confirmed that hardly any psychometric properties were compromised in relation to the 127-item version, suggesting that it is a beneficial measure for ease of use in practice. As a result, this version is the most routinely used in clinical practice today. The measure is copyrighted and available to buy – therefore, full access to the measure is not available – however, a sample of the items is provided for information below; see Figure 6.1 (Barkham et al., 1996).

Once completed by the service user, the total IIP-32 score can be calculated, alongside the eight factors which are: hard to be assertive, hard to be sociable, hard to be supportive, too dependent, too caring, too aggressive, hard to be involved and too open. The outcomes from the questionnaire can be discussed within the assessment with the service user, to see if it corroborates with what

Part I. The following are things you find hard to do with other people.

It is hard for me to:	(not at all)				(extremely)
1. trust other people.	0	1	2	3	4
2. say "no" to other people.	0	1	2	3	4
3. join in on groups.	0	1	2	3	4
4. keep things private from other people.	0	1	2	3	4
5. let other people know what I want.	0	1	2	3	4
6. tell a person to stop bothering me.	0	1	2	3	4

Figure 6.1 Example of IIP-32.

they think of themselves and where some of the difficulties lie within their relationships with others. On completion of the same scale again at the end of the contract of sessions, the outcome scores can be compared, to see if any improvements in such areas of difficulty have occurred (through a reduction of scores).

The Personality Structure Questionnaire

The Personality Structure Questionnaire is a self-report measure, constructed as a tool to assess the individual's experience of personality integration and based upon Ryle's Multiple Self-States Model (MSSM, 1997). The MSSM proposes that adverse early environments are often associated not just with the development of harmful reciprocal roles, but also with a lack of opportunity to develop the self-regulatory and self-reflective capacities needed to smoothly transition from one Reciprocal Role Procedure (RRP) to another. In addition, such environments will often necessitate the use of dissociation as a coping strategy, and this also has the capacity to result in a fragmented and discontinuous sense of self, whereby the individual will experience changes in mood, behaviour and personality as confusing, abrupt and starkly differentiated.

CAT aims to support the increased integration of different elements of the self and hypothesises a continuum from more to less integration along which we all sit. At one end, it is suggested, lie those of us with a more integrated sense of self. At this end of the continuum, we would expect to find that we experience ourselves as more or less the same across different situations, and generally are able to smoothly and flexibly move between different roles as the situation calls for it. It has been argued that those of us who have experienced a more adverse early environment, where the RRPs are harmful in nature, and there have not been the emotional resources available to support a wide variety of flexibly used roles, may sit a little further along this continuum (Ryle refers here to those with a diagnosis of borderline personality disorder, BPD). At the opposite end of the hypothetical continuum sit those of us who have needed to employ dissociation to a much greater degree in order to survive early experiences – this would refer to those diagnosed with dissociative identity disorder (DID), where different parts of the self (or 'alters', as they are sometimes known) can exist completely separately from one another.

As such, Ryle proposed the use of a measure that would give an indication of the degree of personality integration throughout CAT. Broadbent et al. (unpublished, as reported in Pollock, et al., 2001) constructed a self-report measure which aimed to measure identity disturbance (the Personality Structure Questionnaire, or PSQ) – this short eight-item measure asks individuals to rate themselves on a continuum from more to less integration across several domains – for example, "I have a stable and unchanging sense of myself" versus "I am so different at different times that I wonder who I really am".

Pollock et al. (2001) have investigated the psychometric properties of the PSQ by adding to Broadbent et al.'s original samples with clinical and non-clinical samples of their own. These were drawn from the general population, CAT practitioners and health authority employees, those attending a CAT clinic and individuals who had a diagnosis of BPD or DID. Using factor analysis, a screen test indicated that one factor accounted for 40.7% of the variance in PSQ scores. In terms of the internal reliability of the measure (the extent to which all items in a test are related to one another, i.e., they are all measuring the same concept or construct), a Cronbach's alpha of 0.59 was found for the eight-item PSQ (this increased to 0.78 with the removal of item 7, which refers to harm towards self/others; as such, they suggest that item 7 could be removed to increase the integrity of the scale). Additionally, within Broadbent et al.'s sample of students and CAT practitioners, test-retest reliability across a six-week time period was correlated at 0.75, which suggests that the constructs the PSQ is measuring are relatively stable across time.

Pollock et al. (2001) also assessed the convergent validity (the degree to which two measures which should measure the same or similar constructs are in fact related) of the PSQ, within samples drawn from the general population, those with a BPD diagnosis and those with a DID diagnosis. Scores on the PSQ were compared to scores from other measures of identity disturbance (i.e., dissociation, multiplicity, clarity of self-concept, sense of coherence and mood variability). PSQ scores were positively correlated with multiplicity, as measured by the Brief Self-Pluralism Scale (BSPS; Altrocchi et al., 1990), mood variability, as measured by the Mood Variability Scale (MVS; Harvey et al., 1989) and dissociation, as measured by the Dissociative Experiences Scale (DES; Berstein & Putnam, 1986). Interestingly however, the PSQ did not show a positive correlation with dissociation (as measured by the DES) within the DID group. Discriminant analysis indicated that the BPD group scored significantly higher on the PSQ and BSPS, whereas the DID group were higher on the measures of dissociation and mood variability scales. The general population sample showed significantly higher scores on measures of identity integrity and lower scores on measures of identity pathology.

Based on these findings, Pollock et al. (2001) conclude that the PSQ is a reliable and valid measure which does reflect multiplicity as described by the MSSM. In terms of the original continuum proposed, we can say that dissociation did appear to increase in a graded manner from the general population through BPD to DID groups; multiplicity did not, however, with those

	1	2	3	4	5	
	Very true	True	May or may not be true	True	Very true	
1. My sense of self is always the same	0	0	0	0	0	How I act or feel is constantly changing
2. The various people in my life see me in much the same way	0	0	0	0	0	The various people in my life have different views of me as if I were not the same person
3. I have a stable and unchanging sense of myself	0	0	0	0	0	I am so different at different times that I wonder who I really am
4. I have no sense of opposed sides to my nature	0	0	0	0	0	I feel I am split between two (or more) ways of being, sharply differentiated from each other

Figure 6.2 Items of the Personality Structure Questionnaire.

diagnosed with DID not showing any more or less multiplicity than the general population. The Personality Structure Questionnaire is free to use and can be accessed online at Sage Publications. An example of the items on the questionnaire can be found in Figure 6.2.

As with the IIP-32, the PSQ is short, does not take long to complete, and total scores can be computed to gain understanding of pre- and post-therapy outcomes. More importantly, given the PSQ items are on continuums, discussion with the service user of the scores provided can allow for useful understanding of their position on each continuum and what this means for them.

The psychotherapy file

The psychotherapy file was born out of Ryle's wish to define the focus of psychotherapy more specifically as well as his conviction that the changes brought about within therapy are best described in cognitive terms. He refers to the need to collaboratively identify the "mental constructions" (Ryle, 1979) that underlie symptoms and leave us unable to change, thus relating the focus of therapy to these constructions. As we now know, Ryle presents these mental constructions as dilemmas ("false dichotomies that restrict the range of choice"), traps (circular patterns of behaviour which appear to confirm the original perception) and snags (Subtle Negative Aspects of Goals; "I want to change, but …"). In her book *Change for the Better*, Wilde-McCormick (2002) also provides a practical chapter highlighting the contents and use of the psychotherapy file in practice.

In his 1979 paper, Ryle explained that the "dilemmas, traps, snag" (DTS) rating method is derived from clinical work as well as his research into repertory grid techniques and psychoanalytic thinking (as he initially mapped psychosexual development to the problematic patterns within the file, although these were later restated in more cognitive terms). Ryle identified six main types of problems in his review of 25 psychotherapy cases treated by himself (four categories of dilemma, as well as traps and snags). He related the first two dilemmas, *distant or in danger* and *dyadic control* (i.e., either controlling or controlled) to psychoanalytic formulations of separation, individuation and basic trust (the oral stage). The next two dilemmas: *must/won't* and *tight control of feelings versus chaos*, he related to the psychoanalytic concepts of autonomy versus shame and doubt (the anal stage). Lastly, *instrumental versus expressive* dilemmas are often experienced in relation to sex roles; consisting of the person feeling forced to choose between strength and sensitivity, these are thought to relate to the oedipal stage. Ryle described traps as the "interpersonal manifestation of intrapsychic processes" (in other words, the acting out of dilemmas *with others*), relating these in particular to the so-called primitive defence mechanisms of splitting and projective identification. Lastly, he argued that snags (commonly related to feared consequences for, or from, a parent or partner) are linked with the psychoanalytic concepts of fantasy, and ego defences against id and super-ego forces.

Ryle (1979) subsequently reported findings from his use of DTS in clinical practice, both in terms of goal setting and progress tracking within time-limited psychotherapy. He described this method as of particular use to psychotherapists working in the psychoanalytic tradition who had not yet achieved a "definition of focus that is fully effective in guiding clinical work, or that is applicable to research into therapeutic effectiveness".

Contents of the psychotherapy file

Arguably the most commonly used psychotherapy file in practice is the diagrammatic version, originally developed by Mark Dunn in 2002. Through maintaining the original prose structure of the traps, dilemma, snags, and self-states list, the content was not compromised. Whilst the early critique of the diagrammatic file suggested that it could be too overwhelming for many service users, it has stood its test of time for over 20 years in terms of its routine use. This version, amongst others (which will be discussed in the next section), is freely available for members both on the Association of Cognitive Analytic Therapy (ACAT) website and in *Reformulation* (the newsletter for ACAT). The diagrammatic psychotherapy file was updated in 2012 (and is classed as Version 5; ACAT, 2012). It is this version which will be discussed and presented here, as it has been developed to minimise the vast amount of information provided in the 2002 version, for ease of use. In addition, the ACAT (2012) version offers a section to understand difficult and unstable states of mind and alters the self-states list to be termed 'different states'.

Figure 6.3 gives an example of the presentation of a trap within the *diagrammatic psychotherapy file*. There are six common trap types in total. The service user should always be guided to cross out or amend the examples provided, to ensure that the traps make sense to their own personal experiences, rather than feeling they have to fit in with traps presented. The six common trap types include: fear of hurting other people; depressed thinking; trying to please (with two examples); avoidance; social isolation; and low self-esteem (with two examples). All traps are rated on a scale of three from 'does not apply' to 'often applies'.

With regards to dilemmas, the diagrammatic psychotherapy file provides examples of frequently experienced false choices, where limited choice feels

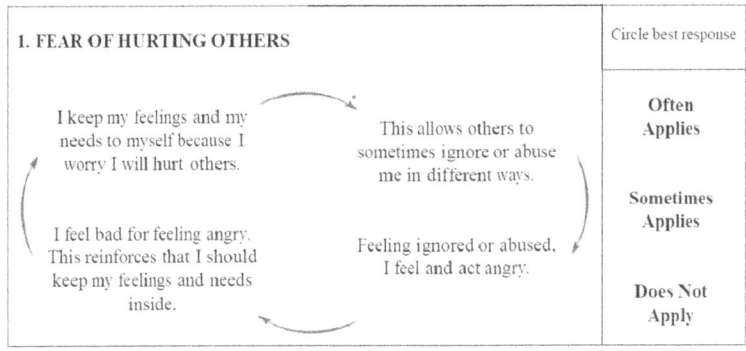

Figure 6.3 Example of a trap from the diagrammatic psychotherapy file (ACAT, 2012).

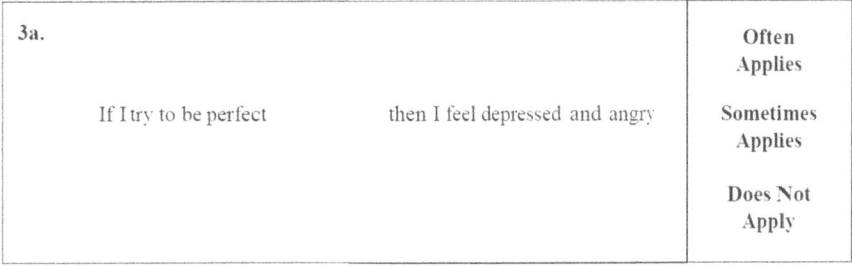

Figure 6.4 Example of a dilemma from the diagrammatic psychotherapy file (ACAT, 2012).

available, and are often experienced as 'either/or' or 'if/then' encounters. Eight of these examples relate to choices about the self, and 11 examples relate to choices in relation to others. Figure 6.4 provides an example of one dilemma, further examples of which include: responsibility; self-sufficiency; upset feelings and clinging, to name a few. Once again, the dilemmas are scored on the same three-point scale as traps.

Two main snags are provided in the psychotherapy file (see Figure 6.5 for example), which highlight the patterns that prevent an individual from getting on with their life (often identified when a person says 'yes but'). Snags are often the most difficult of patterns to identify and to challenge within therapy, as they are often experienced with a strong feeling of guilt should an alternate option be taken. As a result of holding themselves back, the person is left with limited experience of pleasure or success that they may have otherwise encountered.

The 'difficult and unstable states of mind' section of version 5 highlights how individuals' states of mind can fluctuate and change in the midst of difficult experiences. It can often be tricky for people to keep track of these changes as they happen quickly and without warning. There are seven questions within

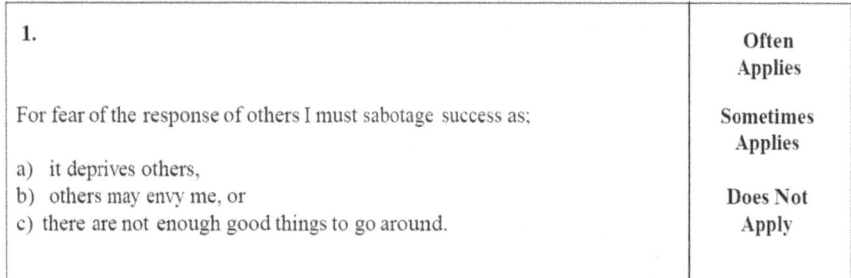

1.	Often Applies
For fear of the response of others I must sabotage success as;	Sometimes Applies
a) it deprives others, b) others may envy me, or c) there are not enough good things to go around.	Does Not Apply

Figure 6.5 Example of a snag from the diagrammatic psychotherapy file (ACAT, 2012).

3.	Often Applies
Other states are accompanied by an emotional blankness, feeling unreal, or feeling muddled.	Sometimes Applies
	Does Not Apply

Figure 6.6 Example of a difficult state of mind from the diagrammatic psychotherapy file (ACAT, 2012).

the psychotherapy file (see Figure 6.6 for an example) which allow individuals to start to recognise whether such unstable states occur and how they feel. These too are scored on the three-point scale. Finally, as a follow-on from this section, the psychotherapy file highlights different states that individuals may identify with. This section differs from the rest, in that it provides a list of possible states, which the service user reads and ticks if they feel the state resonates with them. Examples of difficult states include feeling bad but soldiering on; coping; clinging, fearing abandonment; hurt and humiliated by others; and frightened of others. There is also space at the end of this section for service users to identify their own states, should they wish to do so.

Karen comments on her memories of completing the Psychotherapy File and how she struggles to recall how it was utilised in therapy. She reflects that if she were to answer the questions again now, her responses might be similar to what they were then, yet she knows how to make changes to prevent the pattern from becoming a repeated problem. Such reflections show inherent personality traits, and how these are consistent over time.

Karen says:

> *It was fine, you had to be very honest with it. I can't remember what happened following it.*

Because I probably always will feel, probably the answer will be a martyr [in relation to are you a brute or a martyr?] because that's the type of person I am but I think ticking them like you're looking inward again, like yeah I do 'cos I'm a bit of a martyr yeah it's so long ago. Feeling fearful of hurting others? But you know I think even if you ask me those questions now, although I've worked on myself, I think I'd be ticking the same answers because it's the makeup of you, you are who you are.

Having a discussion with the service user about their responses to the psychotherapy file is important to understand some of the key areas they highlighted as being present for them, particularly to see if these fit with the early understandings the therapist and service user have spoken about within the assessment. Further consideration of how the psychotherapy file is discussed within therapy can be found within Chapter 7.

Adaptations to the psychotherapy file

Often, the version of the psychotherapy file used is based on the therapist's preference with regards to ease of use for service users. As stated above, the *diagrammatic psychotherapy file* (ACAT, 2012) is generally most readily used due to its layout, visual benefits and its reduction in size since the original version. Despite this, there is a dearth of literature to determine the benefits of the psychotherapy file's use in practice and whether or not service users and the therapist find it a useful tool. When reflecting on our own experiences in therapy, we too tend to use it in different ways at different times, either as a tool for discussion within the early reformulatory sessions, to consolidate and evidence already highlighted patterns or as a means of identifying patterns when both service user and therapist feel stuck within their identification.

Despite the lack of evidence base for the use of the file, over recent years, there have been several adaptations made to meet the needs of differing service user groups. The complexity of the file has for a long time been deemed an issue by CAT practitioners, and thus means to make it simpler have been attempted. An early effort by Morris (1995) aimed to create a one-sheet file for service users to complete. Despite the value of this consideration, it does not appear to have been widely incorporated into CAT practice. Similarly in 2006, King developed a 'pull out' shortened version of the file, yet once again, the extent of its usage has been limited.

The need for adapted psychotherapy files has been recognised for the learning disability population and for younger people. Jenaway (2017) collected feedback from teenage service users with regards to how easy the psychotherapy file was to fill in. With nine responses, an average of 7.7 was obtained from a scale of 0–10 where 0 was difficult and 10 was easy. Jenaway (2017) created an adapted version (available on the ACAT website) which is gender neutral, provides statements for identification (rather than multiple choice options) and allows for recognition of positive patterns, rather than solely negative ones.

Despite these brief adaptations made to the psychotherapy file, little else exists in the literature to suggest alternate forms of the file. On reflection, there is vital need for research into the psychotherapy file, particularly to look at the creation of culturally appropriate versions, and given the increase of online therapy, an electronic version of the psychotherapy file would be extremely valuable for ease of completion.

Conclusion

Using objective measures within any therapy can be classed as gold standard, in order to gain useful, impartial information about the service user's wellbeing, both before and after a contract of therapy. In CAT, the personality structure questionnaire and inventory of interpersonal problems are useful, additional measures to be used in conjunction with standard objective measures adopted in services. The psychotherapy file aids understanding of the service user's problematic patterns and is recommended as a tool to be used within the assessment process, followed by discussion within therapy by the service user and therapist to support early mapping.

References

Alden, L. E., Wiggins, J. S. & Pincus, A. L. (1990). Construction of circumplex scales for the Inventory of Interpersonal Problems. *Journal of Personality Assessment*, 55, 521–536. https://doi.org/10.1080/00223891.1990.9674088

Altrocchi, J., McReynolds, P. & House, C. (1990). Self-pluralism as a proposed contributing cause of multiple personality disorder. Poster session at Seventh International Congerence on Multiple Personality Disorder and Dissociation. Chicago.

Association of Cognitive Analytic Therapy (ACAT). (2012). *Updated version of the Psychotherapy File*. CAT Tools. https://www.acat.me.uk/

Barkham, M., Hardy, G. E. & Startup, M. (1996). The IIP-32: A Short Version of the Inventory of Interpersonal Problems. *British Journal of Clinical Psychology*, 35, 21–35. https://doi.org/10.1111/j.2044-8260.1996.tb01159.x

Berstein, E. & Putnam, F. W., (1986). Development, reliability and validity of a dissociation scale. *Journal of Nervous and Mental Disease*, 174, 727–735. https://doi.org/10.1097/00005053-198612000-00004

Dunn, M. (2002). Diagrammatic Psychotherapy File. *Reformulation*, Spring, p.17.

Harvey, P. D., Greenberg, B. R. & Seaper, M. R. (1989). The Affective Lability Scales: Development, reliability and validity. *Journal of Clinical Psychology*, 45, 786–796. https://doi.org/10.1002/1097-4679(198909)45:5%3C786::AID-JCLP2270450515%3E3.0.CO:2-P

Horowitz, L. M. (1979). On the cognitive structure of interpersonal problems treated in psychotherapy. *Journal of Consulting and Clinical Psychology*, 46, 5–15. https://psycnet.apa.org/doi/10.1037/0022-006X.47.1.5

Horowitz, L.M., Rosenberg, S. E., Baer, B. A., Ureno, G. & Villasenor, V. S. (1988). Inventory of Interpersonal Problems: Psychometric properties and clinical applications. *Journal of Consulting and Clinical Psychology*, 56, 885–892. https://psycnet.apa.org/doi/10.1037/0022-006X.56.6.885

Jenaway, A. (2017). An Alternate Psychotherapy File. *Reformulation*, Winter, p. 48.

King, R. (2006). Pull-out Section: The Psychotherapy File. *Reformulation*, Summer issue, pp 7–14.

Morris, P. (1995). See-it-at-a-glance Psychotherapy File, *ACAT Newsletter*, February issue, p 1.

Pollock, P.H., Broadbent, M., Clarke, S., Dorrian, A., & Ryle, A. (2001). Personality Structure Questionnaire (PSQ): A measure of the multiple self states model of identity disturbance in cognitive analytic therapy. *Clinical Psychology & Psychotherapy*, 8 (1), 59–72. https://doi.org/10.1002/cpp.250

Ryle, A. (1979). The focus in brief interpretive psychotherapy: Dilemma, traps and snags as target problems. *British Journal of Psychiatry*, 134, 46–54. https://psycnet. apa.org/doi/10.1192/bjp.134.1.46

Ryle, A. (1997). *Cognitive Analytic Therapy and Borderline Personality Disorder: The Model and the Method*. Wiley.

Wilde-McCormick, E. (2002). *Change for the Better*. Sage.

7 Cognitive Analytic Therapy assessment

Introduction

Now that we have considered some of the main assessment tools and measures for CAT, we can begin to think about what a CAT assessment may involve. It is worth noting that as a practitioner starting out in CAT, you may already have a wealth of transferrable skills in psychological assessment that you can use within a CAT assessment. The CAT assessment is not vastly different to how we would go about completing a more generic psychological assessment, but there are some subtle and important differences that are helpful to take into consideration, in order to gather pertinent information to begin to work together towards reformulation.

In order to set the context of a general psychological assessment, the importance of a trauma-informed stance will be considered initially. Following this, the main attributes of a generic 'psychological assessment' will be reviewed, considering the verbal and non-verbal aspects of an assessment, and what information is helpful to gather. From here, the nuances of a CAT assessment will be discussed, including taking a relational stance to assessment, how to ask questions, and the practical aspects of using the psychotherapy file and objective measures in sessions.

Trauma-informed assessment in CAT

The extent to which difficult early experiences (including abuse and other relational traumas) are explicitly discussed in a psychological assessment is likely to vary between approaches. Whilst previous traumas of many varieties are usually highly relevant to relational patterns and procedures in the here and now, we argue that a trauma-informed approach to assessment is crucial in minimising the risk of re-traumatisation. Upon seeing a new service user for assessment, we may or may not know about their trauma history. Sometimes this might be outlined in previous notes or the referral letter; however on other occasions we may be completely 'blind' to a trauma history. This demonstrates the need to employ a trauma-informed approach to CAT assessment as a 'universal precaution' – because we never know what someone may have experienced

DOI: 10.4324/9781003308256-7

in the past or may be experiencing currently. Trauma-informed care seeks to *realise* the impact and *recognise* the signs of trauma, to *respond* by integrating this understanding into practice and, ultimately, to *resist* the re-traumatisation of individuals we work with (the four Rs; Substance Abuse and Mental Health Services Administration, SAMHSA, 2014).

The principles of trauma-informed care include, amongst others, a focus upon the importance of (physical and psychological) safety, collaboration and choice. These principles seek to redress, or at the very least avoid replicating, the power imbalances that are so inextricably tied to experiences of trauma. So how may we consider CAT assessment through the lens of these principles? We hope that a foundation of transparency and empowerment has begun to be fostered through conversations around informed consent to assessment and treatment (as outlined in Chapter 5). This transparency provides the bedrock for a trusting therapeutic relationship and helps to embed a sense of safety, as the service user knows broadly what to expect from therapy, what it will entail, what the risks are, and, perhaps most importantly, has been empowered to make a choice about whether this is the right approach for them, at the right time, with the right therapist. As far as possible, preferences should be explored and service users should be offered choice regarding the practical elements of assessment sessions – this might include, for example, choice around the venue for the sessions and the timing of appointments. This would also include choices about whether and when they feel able to name or explore previous trauma. The practice of 'routine enquiry' regarding experiences of childhood adversity is explicitly encouraged within mental health services; to ask this question in a truly trauma-informed manner, however, is to ensure that service users feel they have the choice to respond in a way that promotes safety first and foremost. Depending on where someone is in their journey, they may not feel able to acknowledge, or even be fully aware of, their experiences as 'traumatic' or abusive. Service users should be reassured that they do not need to give any further details regarding their experiences at this stage, should they prefer not to. The intention here is not to 'silence' but to support the service user to remain within their window of tolerance, and to leave the door open for this to be returned to in more depth later, should they wish to.

Service users should never be pressured to share more of their story than they are ready to within an assessment, and as such, this may leave us with a dilemma: can we fully reformulate without a shared recognition of key experiences in the service user's life? In such a situation, it may be that we reach a collaborative decision that an approach other than CAT may be indicated – it may be, for instance, that 'stage 1' safety and stabilisation work (Herman, 2015) would be more appropriate as an initial offer. However, it may also be possible to proceed with the assessment in a manner and pace which allow the service user to remain within their window of tolerance, giving voice to what they feel able to and collaboratively settling on a focus for the work which feels to be within their zone of proximal development (ZPD, Vygotsky, 1978). This is of course a nuanced judgement call, and one best discussed with an experienced supervisor; however, we would not seek to unilaterally exclude individuals at different stages in their trauma journey from a potentially helpful therapy. The themes of historical experiences are often evident within here-and-now patterns and can be acknowledged in such a way that is bearable for the service user whilst actively resisting re-traumatisation.

Working in a trauma-informed way also means we see the patterns that have developed as survival strategies used to help make the unbearable bearable and to stay alive. This allows us to recognise the ingenuity and resilience of the human spirit in the face of trauma and to honour patterns which have kept us safe and provided a way of coping with circumstances at that time. The use of language here is so important – oftentimes you will see references in psychological therapy textbooks to 'dysfunctional beliefs and behaviours', 'maladaptive coping strategies', 'primitive defence mechanisms' and 'problem procedures' (CAT is not immune to this!). Whilst it may be the case that strategies developed to survive earlier trauma are no longer needed in the here and now, and in fact are causing problems of their own, a compassionate approach to psychotherapy must begin from a place of validating the origin and the necessity of these patterns in earlier life.

Andrew speaks to how hard it was for him to attend the psychological assessment, how uncomfortable it felt in sharing his story with the therapist, yet he felt the need to attend for the sake of his family.

Andrew says:

> *At the time I didn't want to let the family down, I didn't want to let my wife and the kids down. It was a part of me didn't wanna be there, didn't wanna be anywhere just wanted everything to stop but I think there was a bigger bit of me that wanted to, it was kind of like yeah this is hard, this is uncomfortable but it's entirely possible that I might feel better at the end of this and also kind of a little bit obstinate so kind of like yeah I've got to [give it a] go so I think that mind set helped.*

The main aspects of a 'psychological assessment'

For the purpose of this chapter, we refer to a psychological assessment as being the 'information gathering' and 'getting to know you' phase of the initial contact with the service user. Often, a psychological assessment is defined as comprising both a clinical interview and cognitive testing; however, here we use the term more loosely, and in particular focus on the 'clinical interview' aspect of assessment. Murphy and Dillon (2011) defined a clinical interview as a 'conversation characterised by respect and mutuality; by immediacy and warm presence; and by emphasis on strengths and potential'.

It is within the clinical interview that the foundations of the therapeutic relationship are built, and time to develop a safe and secure environment for the service user is one of the main aims of a psychological assessment. Alongside this, additional aims are also at the forefront of the therapist's mind, including: gaining an understanding of the service user's difficulty and how it impacts currently upon their life; determining whether or not therapy is suitable at this point in time and taking into consideration the service user's life history enough to begin to inform a psychological formulation (Sommers-Flanagan, Zeleke, & Hood, 2015).

A psychological assessment is multi-faceted within its approach and initially the process can be complex for a beginner therapist to navigate. Alongside the practical aspects of how to create a comfortable clinical environment, the clinician also needs to consider their own interviewing skills and both verbal and non-verbal information that is being presented to them within the room. We will consider each of these factors in turn.

Setting up the assessment room

Before welcoming the service user into the assessment, it is important you actively attend to the room in which you are going to be seeing the service user in. Do you have a room available where you can consistently see the service user each week? Is the room well lit? Does it have a comfortable temperature (e.g., not too hot or cold)? Is it soundproof? Does it have matching height chairs (to avoid any power imbalance), and how are you going to set these chairs out in the room? Do you have a small coffee table available for use when completing any shared documents? Are there tissues to hand and water available if the service user needs them? Is there a clock that is easily in sight for both the clinician and the service user? Each of these factors on their own may seem insignificant, but together they form what has been referred to as the 'therapeutic frame' (Cherry & Gold, 1989), and they are key in beginning to develop an environment in which the service user feels safe.

The therapist's interviewing skills

It is, however, not only the environment that helps the service user to feel comfortable. The therapist's persona and ability to engage the service user are also key in developing the therapeutic relationship. Personal warmth, attentiveness, listening skills, empathy and the use of open-ended questions are all key clinical skills a therapist requires within the relationship. Providing detailed, clear and concise information within the introductions – including that of your own role, what to expect of the assessment, how long the session will last, and what will happen thereafter – is also a useful starting point. Attending an initial assessment can be daunting for the service user, and it is essential to provide them with the knowledge that they have to share only what they feel able and that they can stop if the assessment feels too much. As mentioned earlier, in line with the principles of trauma-informed care, the service user needs to be offered full information about what to expect in order to truly gain informed consent. Therefore, providing the service user with as much information as possible with regards to the assessment, highlighting the importance of collaboration within the therapeutic relationship and clearly discussing confidentiality is a central starting point to all assessments.

What to ask?

Where the assessment begins in terms of information gathering is often down to personal choice of the therapist. Some start with early life experiences and work towards the present day. Whereas others start with what is happening for the service user now, and once a full understanding of the difficulties has been gained, the therapist goes back over to find out more about the service user's history. Irrespective of the psychological model to be used, there is key information that needs to be covered within the assessment, in order to begin to understand the service user holistically. Some therapists leave the starting point open to the service user, by using more open-ended questions such as, Where would you like to start today? or What brings you here today?

Often, therapists use the 5Ps of Cognitive Behavioural formulation to structure their assessment (Dudley & Kuyken, 2006). This would include gathering information about the service user's *presenting issues* (e.g., current difficulties and how they are impacting on the service user's life), *precipitating factors* (e.g., what led to/triggered the current presenting issues), *perpetuating factors* (e.g., what keeps the current difficulties going/maintains them), *predisposing factors* (e.g., historical factors in the service user's life that increased their vulnerability to the presenting issue) and *protective factors* (the person's resilience and strengths which maintain their emotional health).

Non-verbal information

It is well accounted for in the literature that only 7 per cent of what we communicate is through spoken words (Mehrabian, 1981). Therefore, the remaining 93 per cent of communication is non-verbal, and particularly shared through our pitch, tone of voice, speed of speech, use of pauses and above all, our body language. With experience, therapists can become attuned to the non-verbal elements of communication, looking out for nuances within body language and shifts in tone of voice, which can indicate potential clues to the service user's thoughts and feelings. Checking in with the service user if the spoken and non-spoken communication appears contradictory can be helpful (e.g., You say you are fine, but I notice you seem a little tearful there?). Similarly, noticing your own emotional reactions to what is said can also be important information, as you may be encountering unspoken feelings within the room (e.g., transference and countertransference).

The main aspects of a CAT assessment

A CAT assessment is likely to cover some of the same ground as a generic psychological assessment; however, the focus within the former integrates the CAT language and frame for therapy, with a noteworthy focus on the service user's relational world. We would understand that the service user's early experiences in life are key in determining their current relational patterns. We might think of these *predisposing factors* in terms of the person's *"relational history"* (Brummer, Cavieres, & Tan, 2024). This perhaps most obviously refers to the quality and nature of their relationships with key others growing up (usually parents/caregivers, but also other family members, and significant adults in their lives). However, it is also important to consider relationships with wider institutions or communities such as religious, social and cultural groups, and the education system. All of these can give rise to key formative experiences in making sense of the self and our position in society. The patterns that emerge from these key early relationships are created to survive those which threaten us and to draw strength from those which nurture us.

Current or recent relationships within adult life may *precipitate* difficulties for the service user because they act as *relational triggers* which echo the roles of past relationships, or at least appear to do so. In exploring this within the CAT assessment, we might ask about romantic relationships and close friendships during adult life, including the ways in which these relationships may have either depleted or nurtured the service user. Relational triggers may also arise in relation to the service user's own children, if they have them, as well as work colleagues and other social contacts.

The *target problem* in CAT can be thought of as the key *presenting* difficulties that the service user has come to therapy for help with. Whilst other models may frame this in terms of a diagnosis (e.g., obsessive compulsive disorder), symptoms (e.g., low mood, self-harming behaviour) or a deficit (e.g., dysfunctional thinking), a CAT assessment defines this through a relational lens, often described as a way of relating that the service user simply has not had the opportunity to learn as yet (e.g., I don't know how to prioritise my own needs). This might be something that the service user is able to articulate right at the start of an assessment, but, as we are more used to talking in terms of symptoms and feeling states, we may need to hold off putting the target problem into (tentative) words until the end of the assessment, when we have enough of an idea about previous and current relational patterns (ideally with as many examples as possible) to summarise these accurately together.

Target problem procedures, then, are seen as the patterns which *perpetuate* the current difficulty – or in other words, 'keep it going'. These are likely to be gleaned by mapping out recent examples of problematic patterns during the assessment sessions or by discussing the TPPs indicated as applying strongly within the psychotherapy file. Typically, these perpetuating factors can involve fears of the potential consequences for self and others of acting differently, beliefs or cognitive biases that give rise to certain behavioural patterns and remain unchallenged and a lack of opportunity to learn other ways of being.

Karen describes here the process of discussing the target problem within the initial assessment with the therapist.

Karen says:

> *From that very first week when the therapist said to me, what is it you want to work on? And I'll say about how I don't wanna feel guilty every time my mom asks me to do something. That I should have done it yesterday and need to do it in my own time and as and when I can. It's that guilt feeling that I'm not good enough for her.*

Healthy reciprocal role procedures or *protective factors* can sometimes feel like an add-on or an afterthought in the typically problem-focussed narratives we often see constructed within mental health services. However, as we shall see below, CAT makes explicit use of the healthy map throughout therapy; noting the service user's existing strengths, resources and healthy relationships, adding to these as therapy progresses.

As already mentioned, there is often an overlap between the 'contents' of a standard psychological assessment and a more specific CAT assessment; however the depth and the way in which questions are asked often differ. CAT's relational lens often seeks to determine information to help begin to develop understanding about the service user's sense of self in relation to others and in relation to themselves. Whilst the following list is not exhaustive, it is hoped that it will provide you with a guide as to what areas to explore within a CAT assessment, using the CAT 5Ps (Brummer et al., 2024) as a structure:

Target Problem (presenting issue):
- What brings you here today?
- How long has your difficulty been going on for?
- What brings you to therapy now?
- Descriptions of difficulty – how does it feel, how long does it last, are there times when you feel better, how would you describe it, who is involved?
- Risk – do you have any thoughts of self-harm or suicide? Do you have any coping strategies that may be risky towards yourself (e.g., drink, drugs)?

Relational Triggers (precipitating factors):
- When did it start?
- What were you doing at the time?
- Were there any other life stressors happening at the time?
- How does it affect your relationship with others?
- How do you feel about yourself?

Relational History (predisposing factors):
- Clinical History questions
- Do you have a birth story? Can you tell me what you know?

- *Can you tell me about your family members? (explore each in detail using relational questioning, e.g., What was mum like as a person? How would you describe her? How was she with you? What did others think of her? If you had to describe her in five words, what would they be?) Where are family members now, what are relationships like currently?*
- *Have you experienced any significant loss/bereavement within your life? How did you cope with this?*
- *Do you have any significant memories from childhood?*
- *Did you experience any trauma or abuse as a child? Has anyone ever behaved towards you in a way that left you feeling uncomfortable? (You do not need to answer this question or provide detail if you do not feel ready)*
- *What was school like growing up? Did you have friends? What were your friendships like? Did you ever experience any bullying?*
- *Who would you go to as a child if you were upset? How were feelings dealt with or responded to in your family?*
- *What happened after you left school? Did you go on to further education or to work?*
- *When did you leave home? What did you do? What was this like for you? How did others react?*
- *Have you experienced any romantic relationships? (explore in detail using relational questioning, e.g., What were these relationships like? How did you feel in relation to the other person? Why did relationships end? What are current relationships like?)*
- *Do you work currently? What is your relationship with work? Do you enjoy the role you do?*
- *Do you have any children? What are these relationships like?*

Target Problem Procedures (perpetuating factors):
- *What keeps you feeling stuck and unable to move forward?*
- *If you could wake up in the morning and a miracle had occurred, what would be different?*
- *When you are feeling like .... What runs through your mind? What would you like to do? How do you go about trying to solve the situation? What happens next?*

Healthy Reciprocal Role Procedures (protective factors):
- *What coping strategies do you have that keep you well?*
- *Is there anyone you currently turn to for support?*
- *Do you have any hobbies or social activities that you enjoy?*
- *How do you look after yourself?*
- *What do you see as your strengths?*
- *What role do religion/spiritual or cultural factors play in your wellbeing?*

Completing a CAT assessment can take time. It is important not to rush this phase of the therapy, as the greater the depth in which the 'getting to know you' part of the approach is completed, the more of a shared understanding is yielded in preparation for the reformulation phase. The first three sessions of the CAT contract are therefore considered part of an extended assessment (often in services, clinicians may see a service user for an initial assessment to determine suitability for therapy and an appropriate choice of approach, which will occur prior to the start of the CAT contract). Within these three sessions, the clinician may explore further with the service user aspects of their relational life, and if needed tools can be used to support the assessment, such as the development of a genogram and/or timeline.

Karen and Andrew share their experiences of the initial sessions in CAT, recognising the benefit of being able to share their life story with the therapist, and how the therapist is beginning to make sense of their experiences. Repeated assessments for service users can be difficult (particularly if they have already shared their life story a number of times already); therefore, it is important to share with the service user the need for you as a therapist to get to know them in their own right, and to hear their experiences from them, rather than other means (e.g. reading previous notes).

Karen says:

I thought it was quite nice because you could go in and sort of offload everything and at first it doesn't feel there's a structure does it because it is just you telling them all about you and all about the history and but then obviously what you don't realise is they are picking up on everything that you're telling them. And as the weeks go on, when you wanna start talking about something else, they can say to you hang on did you not say… kind of like bringing you back into the moment. Because very quickly you realise that they are knowing more about you than you think you've shared. So, they can see things in you that you can't see, and then when they mention it, you think oh she's right I do, do that. Yeah, I am guilty of doing that but that's good because oh you feel as though they're really studying you and it's a good feeling. Because they're telling you what, what you need to know really and making you more self-aware of yourself.

Andrew says:

… but the assessment I remember getting annoyed in that because you give your story and it's not the first therapy and you have to give this story to each one and I know they have to hear it, but you kind of want to get started with this inside I don't want to have to offload all this again because I've already done it so many times. It's boring. And she was very good at calming me down when I didn't realise I was getting annoyed, and you know I was thinking I'm getting upset but you know it wasn't I was getting annoyed. So

first that was I think because it was an awful lot of offloading the first week. That was the first one was like, well, do I want to go back because, you know, I've done this so many times and nothing's working. And, you know, benefit of the doubt would go back and to the second week. But yeah, she would pick up on things that I would think were quite trivial. You know there will be the big things, the bits that I've thought were just affecting why I am like this. And she'd say 'well what about this?' and she was very good at not saying anything, so she would just sit there, and she would fill the silence and that's when she started going into it and it was like 'ohh right'. Oh, she's picked up on something I've not even noticed, but is true.

Attachment theory

As yet, we haven't considered attachment theory too much as an underpinning or integrative part of the evidence base of the CAT model. Generally, in the development of the model, the concept of attachment was limited; it is a theory that needs to be considered, however, particularly as CAT is solidly a relational approach in nature. Jellema (1999) introduced the specific need to include attachment theory, given its similarities to the key areas of the CAT model. In particular, Jellema (1999) spoke of the importance of attachment needs in human motivation of survival, for example, to ensure we feel safe, secure and out of danger. In addition, attachment alongside CAT sees the importance of early experiences in developing the longer-term ways in which we engage with others (e.g., in CAT the reciprocal role procedures) and why abusive relationships can persist (e.g., in destructive relationships where the 'secure base' is at the same time the 'dangerous stressor': the greater the stress from the secure base, the greater the pull back to that figure).

We decided to introduce attachment theory at this point in particular, as it fundamentally underpins a CAT assessment. The early sessions are not only about engaging the service user through asking questions to gather an in-depth understanding about their difficulties and life history, but primarily about beginning to develop a therapeutic relationship. We have already spoken about safety, security and trust as part of a trauma-informed assessment. These are key attachment principles and central in developing a therapeutic relationship which is collaborative, open and in confidence, and which in time can offer a 'corrective, emotional experience' (Jellema, 1999). Focussing on these attachment principles early on within the therapeutic contact has been found to strengthen the working alliance and lower the risk of the service user prematurely ending therapy (Kietaibl, 2012).

In addition, the focus on attachment in the therapeutic relationship should not only be through considering the service user's potential attachment styles and how they may relate to the therapist, but also for the therapist to understand their own attachment style and what they may bring into the room. In doing so, the therapist can reflect more openly in supervision as to what interactions they feel belong to themselves and what belongs to the service user.

It has been highlighted that therapists with secure attachment styles may be able to handle therapeutic ruptures more easily (Meyer et al., 2001).

Karen says:

> *She highlighted it the first day and she said one of my concerns is that I think kind of at the first session having listened to you and see that there is, you do tend to attach, and I do, there's no denying that. So, she highlighted that pretty quick and that was my inner determination to prove her wrong. It was about 20 weeks in all.*

Objective measures

As discussed in Chapter 6, we use objective measures as therapists to measure change. We often talk about three different types of change: subjective (the service user's view), clinical (the therapist's view) and objective (that provided by a questionnaire). In order to gain an objective view of change, we need the service user to complete objective measures before therapy starts and once it comes to an end. As discussed in Chapter 6, the two main objective measures used in CAT are the Inventory of Interpersonal Problems (IIP, Horowitz et al., 1988) and the Personality Structure Questionnaire (PSQ, Pollock et al., 2001).

The IIP is useful on an additional level at the start of therapy to indicate the main areas of difficulties in relationships that the service user finds 'too hard to do'. The PSQ is a suitable tool to help address problems to be targeted during CAT, and in particular is able to assess 'multiplicity', the assumption that identity comprises multiple selves, which can be more or less integrated, adaptive, fluid, coherent and consistent (Rowan, 1990).

Asking the service user to take home the measures at the end of the first session, or alternatively sending them out with the initial appointment letter for completion prior to the first session, is a good starting point. Spending time with the service user to discuss areas they have highlighted as being the most difficult to currently complete within the IIP will aid in the gathering of information about the target problem. Here, the service user and therapist can work together collaboratively, to really get a sense of what the service user finds too difficult to do. Additionally, the PSQ provides helpful information for the therapist and service user to spend time considering how the service user finds themselves as a 'constant' in different settings, or whether they experience a more variable sense of self made up of distinct parts. Each one of these outcome measures is easy to complete and to score. The scores can then be compared across different time points (e.g., before and after therapy) to determine any reduction and thus improvement in wellbeing. Individual responses to questions can be used as points of discussion for the therapist to gather more information from the service user. Having such discussions within a session can highlight the importance of completing the measures to the service user, as often all too readily in clinical practice they can be asked to complete forms and questionnaires on which they receive no feedback.

The use of the psychotherapy file

The psychotherapy file is a really helpful tool to use as part of the assessment in order to gain further information from the service user about their problematic patterns. We have already considered its contents in Chapter 6; therefore, here we contemplate how and when to use the tool within the assessment phase.

It is often useful to provide dedicated time at the end of the initial or second session to explain the psychotherapy file fully to the service user. It is a large document and could feel overwhelming for a service user if provided with no explanation; therefore, we would always recommend giving it to the service user within the early contract of CAT, once a therapeutic relationship has begun to be established. Prior to the session, choose the version of the psychotherapy file (see Chapter 6 for more information) that you feel the service user would benefit most from.

You may have already explained to the service user about problematic procedures, but if not, now is the time to do so. The following is a script that you may wish to use or adapt to be your own, to introduce the psychotherapy file to the service user:

'This is a long questionnaire that I would like you to take home to complete over the next week, at your own leisure. You don't have to complete it all in one go; you may wish to break it down into sections and complete some parts each day. The psychotherapy file is broken down into three different types of problematic patterns that we can all get caught up within at times – they are called Traps, which are often also thought of as vicious circles; Dilemmas, our either/or options – and Snags, which are our 'yes, but' patterns.

The file gives you examples of each of these different types of problematic patterns to work through. Your job is to rate how much or little each pattern applies to you (e.g., often applies, sometimes applies or does not apply). The file is only there to provide examples, we are not in any way trying to fit you into these patterns that are provided.'

Provide an example of a trap from the Psychotherapy file here. Handy hint... If you already have an idea of what one of your service user's patterns could be, use this one to talk through your example (e.g., if the service user has spoken about feeling as though they worry about upsetting others and therefore always strive to do what others want, choose the trying-to-please trap). Using an example the service user can relate to will make it more meaningful to them, and thus they are more likely to complete the file.

'This file is yours to keep, and therefore if parts of the patterns that are provided do not make sense to you or relate to you, then cross parts out and add in *information of your own, so it feels more like your own. There may be some patterns that you find really feel like yours and others that don't relate to you at all. This is absolutely fine.*

The difficult and unstable states of mind section also allows you to read through different examples and rate yourself on a scale of often applies, sometimes applies and does not apply. This section aims to look at how our states of mind may feel different and difficult at times.

Finally, the different states section looks at how we feel about ourselves and how the world can change in sudden and confusing ways for some people. Different examples of these states are provided, and it's your job to read through them and put a tick next to the ones (if any) you experience, and there is space for you to add in any that you experience that may not be listed. If you could complete the file over the next week, we can come back together in the next session to discuss what you have written. However, if you go away and find it's too difficult or you struggle to make sense of it, please do not worry. Just leave it and we can discuss it further together next time.'

At the start of the next session, it is worth checking in on how the service user found the psychotherapy file, and to talk through some of the patterns that strongly resonated with them. The way in which the service user responds to this piece of homework is also a helpful piece of information for the therapist (remember how much we get from non-verbal information). It is worth thinking through with the service user their experience of completing the file, and if any different presentations are noted (e.g., forgotten homework, all patterns being rated as strongly applies, all patterns being rated as does not apply). We generally tend to discuss only the patterns that the service user has rated as 'often applies' to them, and curiously ask for examples of these patterns from the here and now, and from early life in childhood. If you are uncertain of how to make sense of the psychotherapy file and how the service user has completed it, gain advice from your supervisor as to how to manage this.

The psychotherapy file is a good way of beginning to notice patterns you may be starting to map out with the service user. It is also a helpful way of corroborating whether or not your own early 'clinical hunches' about problematic patterns match what the service user is identifying. It can be a useful way of leading into mapping and moving into the reformulation phase of therapy.

The healthy map

People naturally seek out psychological therapy when something is 'wrong', and they are struggling (if everything was just fine, they would likely have little reason to attend) – and so it stands to reason that they will be expecting to talk about this. Often, we as therapists will also be expecting to *ask* about this. However, our service users also come to us with their unique talents, interests, skills and strengths, and we do them and the therapy, a huge disservice if we do not attend to these. The healthy map (just like the naming of the 'protective factors') should not be an afterthought but rather should be part of the dialogue from the very beginning of therapy. This of course does not mean that we should aim to have a healthy map fully constructed within the first few assessment sessions – rather that we should carefully listen out for opportunities to ask about and notice the service user's healthy relationships or relational patterns (with themselves or others), their strengths and their survival strategies throughout. As we do this, it is also important to recognise that many of us struggle to identify our strengths, we may feel suspicious of someone who appears to 'compliment' us, or even feel invalidated if the positives are highlighted before the difficulties are properly attended to. For this reason, it is best to be tentative and curious when reflecting upon the service user's strengths early on in therapy – as the sessions progress and you get to know your service user in more depth, you will gain a better sense of how highlighting healthy parts will be received. Likewise, it can be helpful to acknowledge with the service user that you are going to be focussing on some of their difficulties and what brought them to therapy, yet this does not discount the fact that they will have many strengths and healthy parts to themselves, and that you will return to these as your discussions progress.

Risk mapping and management

All psychotherapy assessments need to focus upon risks, and CAT is no different – here we shall briefly consider the main areas of risk assessment to be covered within a CAT assessment and make some suggestions as to how the CAT model can assist in collaboratively recognising and managing these. Risks broadly fall within the categories of 'risks to self' and 'risks to other' and can be some of the most challenging issues to navigate within a psychological therapy relationship.

In relation to the risks posed by suicidality, we would recommend careful consideration and clinical judgement (supported by supervision) on a case-by-case basis. Whilst a period of acute suicidality is unlikely to be the best time to embark upon a challenging episode of psychological therapy – we would argue that it is important not to arbitrarily exclude from a potentially helpful intervention those who struggle with chronic feelings of suicidality. It will be important to enquire within the assessment about past and current suicidal thoughts, plans, actions and protective factors (including the typical antecedents: what factors tend to exacerbate these impulses and what factors tend to reduce them). It is possible to construct a mini-formulation of risk using the CAT 5Ps framework (Brummer et al., 2024) and to generate a shared plan of what the service user can do to manage risk, what others around them can do, and what services can do.

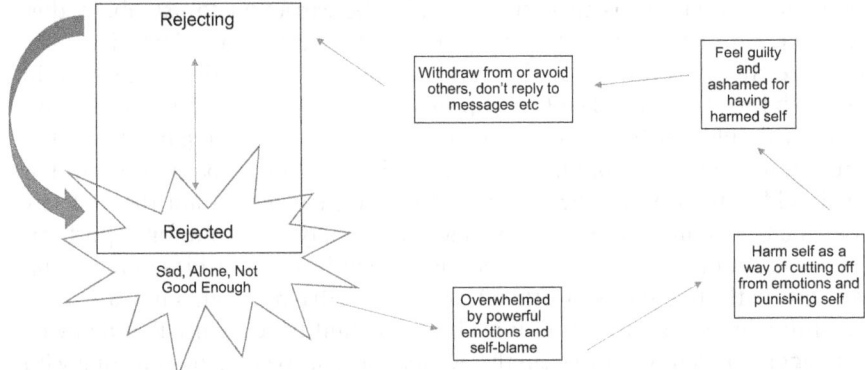

Figure 7.1 Example of a risk-related procedure.

Whilst it is outside the scope of this text to detail the intricacies of risk assessment, we would like to attend to the ways that CAT mapping can help make sense of risk-associated patterns. In our experience, risk-related procedures are often associated with escape from the area of 'core pain' – the most unbearable and feared 'place' on the map (see Chapter 5 for further definition). Suicide might be seen as the 'ultimate escape' from this place, but other coping behaviours, which are potentially harmful to the self, may also feature (e.g., alcohol and drug misuse, cutting/burning/scratching, risky sexual behaviour and self-starvation). If the service user is willing to do so, jointly mapping out a recent example of a time when the risk to self increased or was acted upon can be useful in exposing the chain of events, thoughts and feelings that typically lead them into this place (see Figure 7.1 for an example of a risk related procedure). Early recognition of the individual function that these suicidal or self-harming thoughts, impulses and behaviours have for the service user can also be useful in identifying less harmful alternatives.

Andrew and Karen share their experiences of discussion of risk within their early sessions with their therapists. They explain the importance of feeling safe and contained within the therapy room, to share their experiences, and how beneficial it was for the therapist to remain calm, not to react in panic, and to be able to think openly with them about a management plan.

Andrew says:

> *You do the score sheets and everything, one of the first questions you know is do you have any thoughts of suicide or self-harm. My answer was always 'yes'. How often? 'All the time'. I'm not going to do something about it. No, it's just I think about that, it's always an option. So probably quite rightly they're like do we need to do an action plan, you know to put one in place. 'No'. So, like with her [therapist] I don't think she did that. When I said to*

her 'you know if this kind of doesn't work then I've got nothing'. But it didn't feel like I had to explain exactly straightaway it was, erm, we will have to put a plan in place. And it's not just move on and that helped. So, like I said, the first one is always kind of no, I don't need help. No, I don't need the crisis. Yes, I have the phone number. It's just this is my reality. Contemplating suicide is always there, it's always an option, it's not necessarily what I will do but it's what keeps me sane. It's my safe place bizarrely enough.

I think she did say 'I have to report this' and yes quite rightly too, but she wasn't … she was so calm throughout and she was like 'you are aware of… that you know that this dictates what I need to do' and I was like 'yeah'. She didn't make a big thing of it whereas some therapists… quite a few therapists would.

So, the trust must have come because she was the first therapist I told that I'd taken an overdose and again there was no alarm bells, there was no nothing and she was like 'who else have you told?' And I was like, 'you're the first person'. She was like 'does your wife know', and I was like 'no'. And we spent sort of that session analysing why I'd done it. And why it was sort of still a thought, you know, for me, it was everything stopped, that was peace was the first time that I've had peace in my life. And it was the peace I craved, not the suicide. Not the not being here, it was the bit beforehand where it was like and it kind of normalised it that it wasn't necessarily a bad thing but it was that peace that I craved and that really helped and that was a powerful session.

Karen says:

You have to be able like to discuss it as well. You have to be able to discuss why you think you want to take your life. And I think it's nice to be able to discuss it without feeling frightened. Like if it's an option and the person might consider it then just explore it but don't be frightened. It's just something that's probably the most natural thing to do.

There are, of course, also times in therapy when you will be alerted to the risk of harm to others. This may be harm from the service user, should they display tendencies towards violence and aggression, or it may be that you become aware of information which suggests others could be at risk of harm from a third party (an example of this is a disclosure of historic child sexual abuse where the alleged perpetrator was not convicted and has ongoing unsupervised access to children).

It will be important within the assessment to enquire about any history of violence and aggression towards others if this information is not already known. There also may be patterns and procedures which are related to states of out-of-control rage. These will be crucial to be aware of. It will be necessary to understand together general de-escalation procedures, service user specific triggers and arousal reduction techniques.

It is of utmost importance that where there is an identified risk of not to harm to others, the therapist uses all the usual safety measures available to them to minimise this risk (for example, avoiding lone working, ensuring the individual is seen within a clinic setting at a time when others are around, the use of personal alarms, sitting nearest the exit, etc.). Ultimately, only the individual therapist can decide (in collaboration with their supervisor) what level of risk they are comfortable working with. Whilst Bion (1961) is widely quoted to have said that "if there aren't two anxious people in the room ... then there was not much point in turning up", we can't *become* a place of safety for our service users if our own threat system is too activated.

It is worth here returning to the example above of disclosures of historic child sexual abuse – in this situation we must be mindful both of our duty of care to the service user and our duty to safeguard others. It is surprisingly common for staff in mental health services to shy away from following up disclosures with enquiries surrounding potential ongoing risk to others. This is understandable on a number of levels – service users can feel conflicted about sharing this information if the perpetrator was a family member, someone in a position of power or authority or if they fear being shamed or not believed. Staff can also feel conflicted about following this up for fear of making the service user feel uncomfortable, for fear or damaging the therapeutic relationship or simply because they are not clear what they could or should do with this information even if it were obtained. Again, whilst it is not within the scope of this text to explore this issue in any depth, we encourage readers to educate themselves on this issue using materials such as The British Psychological Society's (2016) *Guidance Document on the Management of Disclosures of Non-recent (Historic) Child Sexual Abuse.*

Conclusion

A CAT assessment is predominantly distinguished by its relational approach. In particular, this includes gathering information from the service user about their own relationships throughout their life with others and themselves, as well as considering the non-verbal information and development of the therapeutic relationship within the room. When completing a CAT assessment, it is imperative to ensure that it is trauma-informed and collaborative. The first three sessions in CAT are defined by developing a further understanding of the service user's presenting problems and history, as well as using outcome measures and the psychotherapy file to further collate useful information. Early mapping can occur within these sessions, to tentatively highlight the beginnings of an SDR, to map risk as well as highlight healthy patterns the service user has. The CAT assessment paves the way for the reformulation process, which will ultimately include mapping and the reformulation letter.

References

Bion, W. R. (1961). *Experiences in Groups*. Basic Books.

British Psychological Society. (2016). *Guidance Document on the Management of Disclosures of Non-Recent (Historic) Child Sexual Abuse*. The BPS.

Brummer, L., Cavieres, M., & Tan, R. (Eds). (2024). *The Oxford Handbook of Cognitive Analytic Therapy*. (online Ed.). Oxford Academic https://doi.org/10.1093/oxfordhb/9780198866572.001.0001

Cherry, E. F. & Gold, S. N. (1989). The therapeutic frame revisited: A contemporary perspective. *Psychotherapy*, 26(2), 162–168. https://psycnet.apa.org/doi/10.1037/h0085415

Dudley, R. & Kuyken, W. (2006). Formulation in Cognitive Behavioural Therapy: There's nothing good or bad, but thinking makes it so. In L. Johnstone & R. Dallos (Eds.), *Formulation in Psychology and Psychotherapy: Making Sense of People's Problems*. (pp. 17–46). Routledge.

Herman, J. L. (2015). *Trauma and Recovery: The Aftermath of Violence—From Domestic Abuse to Political Terror*. Basic Books.

Horowitz, L. M., Rosenberg, S. E., Baer, B. A., Ureño, G., & Villaseñor, V. S. (1988). Inventory of interpersonal problems: Psychometric properties and clinical applications. *Journal of Consulting and Clinical Psychology*, 56(6), 885–892. https://psycnet.apa.org/doi/10.1037/0022-006X.56.6.885

Jellema, A. (1999). Cognitive Analytic Therapy: Developing its theory and practice via attachment theory. *Clinical Psychology and Psychotherapy*, 6(1), 16–28. https://doi.org/10.1002/(SICI)1099-0879(199902)6:1%3C16::AID-CPP182%3E3.0.CO;2-N

Kietaibl, C. M. (2012). A review of attachment and its relationship to the working alliance. *Canadian Journal of Counselling and Psychotherapy*, 46(2), 122–140. ISSN 0826-3893

Mehrabian, A. (1981). *Silent Messages: Implicit Communication of Emotions and Attitudes*. Wadsworth.

Meyer, B., Pilkonis, P. A., Proietti, J. M., Heape, C. L., & Eagan, M. (2001). Attachment styles and personality disorders as predictors of symptom course. *Journal of Personality Disorders*, 15(5), 371–389. https://doi.org/10.1521/pedi.15.5.371.19200

Murphy, B. C. & Dillon, C. (2011). *Interviewing in Action in a Multicultural World*. (4th Ed). Brookes/Cole.

Pollock, P. H., Broadbent, M., Clarke, S., Dorrian, A. & Ryle, A. (2001). The Personality Structure Questionnaire (PSQ): A measure of the multiple self states model of identity disturbance in Cognitive Analytic Therapy. *Clinical Psychology and Psychotherapy*, 8, 59–72.

Rowan, J. (1990). *Subpersonalities: The People Inside Us*. Routledge.

SAMHSA. (2014). *SAMHSA's Concept for Trauma and Guidance for a Trauma Informed Approach*. https://store.samhsa.gov/product/SAMHSA-s-Concept-of-Trauma-and-Guidance-for-a-Trauma-Informed-Approach/SMA14-4884

Sommers-Flanagan, J., Zeleke, W., & Hood, M. H. (2015). Clinical Interview. In S. Lilienfeld & R. L. Cautin (Eds.), *The Encyclopaedia of Clinical Psychology*. Wiley.

Vygotsky, L. S. (1978). *Mind in Society: The Development of Higher Psychological Processes*. Harvard University Press.

8   The reformulation letter

Introduction

At the end of the initial Cognitive Analytic Therapy (CAT) assessment sessions, the process of writing the reformulation letter (RL) begins. Sharing the RL marks a point in therapy where the 'sense making' of the service user's difficulties is embarked upon. Whilst early mapping may have occurred already, the RL signifies a prose (re)telling of the service user's story. This chapter aims to guide the developing CAT practitioner through the course of writing the letter, the therapist's emotional investment during writing, the general structure and content of the letter and differing ways of writing and sharing the letter in therapy. Andrew shares his reformulation letter at the end of the chapter.

How do I start to write the letter?

Knowing what to write and how to write an RL can often be a daunting process. Even the most experienced practitioners can find themselves stuck at the start of writing. Sitting at a computer screen with a blank word document, you can often find your mind whirring with conversations you have had in therapy so far, key experiences the service user has encountered or early reciprocal roles and target problem procedures you have begun to identify. It may feel overwhelming wondering where to start, and, in reality, there is no right or wrong way to begin. In time, most practitioners find their own style, their own flow, and their own process of writing the letter.

Having said that, we can share that there are some useful tips when you come to write your RL. Engaging in writing the letter is a practice that takes time, effort and emotional involvement. It is best to book out protected time in your diary where you won't be interrupted and where you can find a quiet space to reflect and begin to write. Wilde McCormick (2008) spoke of the importance of "spending time in inner dialogue with your inner writer" when putting pen to paper. In order to do this, you really need to have the time and space to re-immerse yourself within the service user's narrative and consider how and what you want to write.

DOI: 10.4324/9781003308256-8

It is useful to use written notes you have made from the assessment, to re-orientate yourself to the service user's experiences and to the key relationships that you are wanting to focus on. You may also review the psychotherapy file (if the service user has completed it at this point) and note patterns that the service user has highlighted as 'always occurring'. Similarly, if early mapping has already begun in sessions, you may want to have the map in front of you as you write, so you can hold in mind some of the relational dynamics that you have already begun to identify. Finally, think about how you have felt in the room with the service user. This often gives a good indication of reciprocal roles and key emotions that are present, as you may want to comment on these later within your letter, with an acknowledgement of how together you may manage difficult situations if they emerge. In holding some of these feelings in mind, you are likely to get in touch with your 'inner writer' and feel freer in writing about how you truly feel.

When beginning to write (whether it be in your own handwriting or on a computer), be aware of and familiar with the general contents of a letter (see section on the contents of the reformulation letter). Use the contents as a guide to writing the letter in narrative form. For us, in reflecting on our own style of writing, we recognised that we both find it easy to start at the beginning and work sequentially through the letter from the beginning to the end. This sounds like a simplistic process but may in fact help with the flow of the narrative and prevent the letter from sounding disjointed. A RL is a very different way of writing. Professional reports are often formal, comprising jargon, and the writer is often mindful of the content and what needs to be shared within the letter. Conversely, RLs always have the service user at the centre of their content and are written directly to them. You have to hold the service user in mind, all the way through writing, and think about how they may receive what you write. Returning to the earlier consideration of being aware of how you feel as you come to write the letter, throughout the process take moments to be mindful of your emotions (e.g., are you scared, excited, stuck, overwhelmed, bored, sad, tired?). Whatever the feeling, take regular opportunities to stop and reflect on whether this remains or changes as you write. You may experience counter-transference of the service user's core pain, and at times within the letter, you may want to share this tentatively with them (e.g., 'in writing this letter I am struck by the sadness I feel in relation to what you have encountered ...'). Alternately, you may be experiencing feelings of your own that are preventing you from being able to think clearly and write.

When immersed in writing, you may at times feel overcome with emotion, whilst at other times you feel you are approaching things differently. You may find that you have to stop yourself and take stock because you haven't reflected as you usually do or have felt detached from what you are writing. This too is useful information, as it may mirror the service user's own strategies of cutting off from emotions or feeling that others don't hold them in mind. Personal experiences of writing reformulation letters can differ from service user to service user, and thus frequent self-reflection is important. There may be several reasons as to why you are reacting the way you are to writing a letter, for example: the service user's personal story may be similar to something you have experienced, you may be getting caught within the dance of a target problem procedure or there may be emotions of your own that are being evoked. Each reaction can impact your own writing style, leaving some letters feeling easy to write and flowing well, whereas others can feel difficult, stilted and as though the words just don't come freely. As CAT practitioners, we find supervision is always invaluable in helping to understand these reactions. We will stress throughout this chapter to *always* take your RL to share in supervision before you share it with the service user. For this part, however, we also want to stress the importance of also taking your *experience* of writing the letter to reflect on in supervision too.

We have our own key memories of times when supervision has helped us to recognise when we were getting caught up within a target problem procedure when writing a letter. On one occasion, Sarah's supervisor fed back, "Sarah, this isn't written like you would normally write one of your letters. There is no emotion within it, and you appear detached and distant from the service user." Supervision was then spent considering why this was the case, and helping Sarah get in touch with the service user's core pain, which had been hidden and avoided within sessions up until that point. In doing so, more emotion was then added to the letter, which in turn enabled the service user to identify that it was safe and 'okay' to name how they really felt. Similarly, Jayne recalls how difficult an early reformulation letter was to write for fear of getting something wrong; supervision helped to recognise that this wasn't just beginner's nerves but an identification with the projection of the part of the service user that was terrified of feeling rubbished or criticised. Stepping out of this stuckness inevitably entailed the recognition that mistakes are human and that modelling the survival of getting things wrong was likely to be more therapeutic than trying to strive for perfection.

The next section considers the general contents of a reformulation letter, its length and key areas to consider. Again, this is by no means a prescriptive 'how-to' of writing, as this would lose the individuality and person-centred nature of the approach.

The contents of the reformulation letter

As we have emphasised already, each reformulation is unique and tailored to the individual. However, there are some key areas which it will be important to consider when deciding what to include in your letter. It is important to clearly state, at an early stage of the letter, that what you are sharing is a draft – finding some way of expressing the tentative nature of the letter is crucial. As therapists we must stay as close as possible to what the service user has told us. Although there will inevitably be a layer of facilitated 'sense making' that we as therapists add to the letter, it is important that the service user owns its contents, that we remain open to hearing that we may have got parts wrong, missed things out, or misinterpreted their words. This is particularly important where a service user's previous experiences may lead them to want to please us or cast us in the light of an 'expert position'. Alongside this, it can be useful to set out a reminder as to the intended purpose of the letter – you will already have discussed this with the service user; preparing to hear an RL can be an anxiety-provoking experience, however, and it can be reassuring to provide a reminder early on in the letter that the intention is to summarise what has been discussed in sessions so far with the aim of agreeing upon a focus for the remainder of the work.

In order to draw the service user's attention back to their 'reason why', it can be useful to briefly summarise what has led them to seek out therapy at this particular time; in other words, what is motivating them to embark upon this challenging journey? If you have a good enough sense of it, you can also refer to what you and the service user understand to be their target problem (TP) and associated aim for therapy. It might not always be completely clear at this stage of therapy, so again, being tentative here is important ("I wonder whether ..."). Additionally, in keeping with the principles of Trauma Informed Care, it can also be helpful to frame the TP in terms of the ways of relating that the service user hasn't yet had a chance to learn (due to their previous experiences). This takes a subtle but important step away from a deficit-based understanding of mental health and presents the aim as a skill that can be learnt, like any other.

As discussed in the previous section, after these important introductory messages have been communicated, usual practice would be to start from the beginning, with the service user's earliest relevant experiences. This will usually include a description of their family of origin and their felt experience of growing up in this relational environment. Key childhood events, relationships and traumatic experiences are named, where relevant, although it is important to bear in mind the service user's zone of proximal development (ZPD) here. On several occasions we have worked with service users who were able to allude to abusive or traumatic early experiences without naming them directly. There can be many very understandable reasons for this: a wish to protect key caregivers, a sense that recognising an experience as abusive will be too painful, or even a lack of clarity in their minds about whether what they experienced was actually abusive or not. It is important to also recognise that trauma memories are often fragmented and can be experienced as jumbled and unclear. In these cases, careful use of clinical judgement and supervision is needed to sensitively word your letter. Naming something that you consider to be abusive as such, when the service user does not think of it in this way for whatever reason, can be damaging. On the other hand, recognising something as harmful, and clearly laying responsibility in the hands of the alleged perpetrator, when the service user blames themselves, can also begin to pave the way to greater self-compassion. A key consideration, regardless of how you choose to word your description of difficult (early) experiences, is the recognition of how the service user survived, honouring what they had to do to cope, even if these same strategies are now causing difficulties. It is important to also start to help the service user think about what they may have learnt from these experiences – what beliefs were resultantly formed about themselves, the world, and others, about how best to cope with relationships, people and feelings. A description of a key event or relationship alone is not enough; the letter must also include a recognition of what this may have been like, felt like or meant to the service user. Again, it is best to use the service user's own words and cultural references wherever possible in making these links; we also need to bear in mind, however, that many service users may not have grown up in an environment with a care-taker who was able to facilitate their emotion recognition capabilities for vari-ous reasons. There may have been no adult around who could help them name and make sense of their feelings. This is where, as a therapist, we might begin to facilitate this recognition by offering up a tentative 'wondering' on how a key event or relationship might have left them feeling. This can then be linked to a hypothesis about what they learned from the relationship/event and, perhaps most importantly, the link can be made with ongoing 'problem procedures' that have been carried through to the current day. We find that italicising key words within the letter to highlight core pain, key reciprocal roles and problem-atic patterns can be helpful to emphasise their importance to the service user.

Whilst some key relationships and life events may clearly relate to the ser-vice user's presenting difficulties and target problem procedures, it can be hard to know how much of their overall life story to include in the letter if there is a lot of potentially relevant information. If the letter goes beyond three pages in length, you might want to reconsider whether any of the information can be condensed or taken out, to aid with maintaining the focus. It will be important to mention any early exits taken in therapy so far in the letter as well as current strengths and resources. We would strongly recommend that you reflect upon and name any patterns that may come up within the therapeutic relationship towards the end of the letter, for example, for a service user with a people-pleasing pattern you might highlight that:

> ...We will need to be alert to any times when these patterns may come up between us – it may be that you will feel pulled into trying to please me at times; for instance, if this happens it will useful for us to notice this and talk about it so that we can create an opportunity to make sense of this and do something different.

Lastly, it is important to mention the ending of the therapy within the reformu-lation letter, both so that this is named and kept in conscious awareness but also so that you can tentatively wonder about any feelings or urges that may emerge for the service user in response to this, based on what you now know about their roles and patterns already. Some CAT practitioners will tend to embed the description of TPPs only within the body of the letter, whereas oth-ers will add an additional sheet after the end of the letter with a numbered list of TPPs as well, for ease of reference.

The sharing of the reformulation letter

Once you have written your RL and taken it to supervision to read, discuss and make any recommended alterations, you are ready to share the letter in therapy. For the therapist, the preparation of writing the letter outside of therapy takes time; within the therapy, the service user too needs preparation in knowing the letter will come. In the initial stages of introducing the service user to the model of CAT, you may have spoken about the use of letters, and directed the service user towards when to expect them. As you work towards session 4 in therapy, again it is important to discuss with the service user when will be best to share the RL. There are a number of considerations that need to be made when planning for the RL session:

- Do you and the service user feel ready for the sharing of the letter? (e.g., is the assessment sufficiently complete? If more time is needed, the letter may be shared in session 5, although be aware of potentially delaying the letter due to your own avoidance!)
- Have you planned time outside of the therapy room to write the letter and take it to supervision?
- Is there a session planned for the week after sharing the letter? (If not and there is a break planned, you may consider together whether to share the letter on the return to therapy. Leaving the service user with the letter without space to discuss it in therapy in the subsequent session can be difficult for them.)

Once you have considered these factors, you can have an open conversation with the service user and agree on the most appropriate session to share the letter.

Within the RL session (session 4/5) it is often useful to open the session with the session number, and a reminder that today had been planned for the sharing of the RL. It is useful to check with the service user how they felt coming to the session knowing that the letter was coming. In a recent session for Sarah, a service user responded "I'm interested in hearing what sense you make of my difficulties and how they are linked with my past experiences".

It is important to ensure that enough time is dedicated to the reading of the RL and with time afterwards to discuss it. Often as therapists we will want to check in on how the last week has been for the service user, which is useful and necessary for them to impart any key experiences first. Being aware of time, and not being pulled into avoiding the letter is also vital. Leaving insufficient time to share and discuss the letter can be problematic and can impact on the experience for the service user in hearing their letter. Hamill et al. (2008) researched the service users' experience of receiving letters in CAT. They found that where the experience was felt to be negative, reasoning for this included: insufficient time for discussion of the letter, lack of accuracy, being handed the letter to read or being told a copy of the letter would be given at a later date.

Ensuring you hold the service user in mind throughout the process of sharing the letter is therefore extremely important to aim to prevent any adverse effects (Newell et al., 2009).

We use the term 'sharing' loosely, as practitioners find their own style in how to facilitate the RL session, but also this may differ between service users, dependent upon their needs. What is important about the term 'sharing' is that it implies a two-way process, for example, to let someone have something that belongs to you. It suggests collaboration, and this relational aspect is at the heart of the RL process. It should always be inclusive of the service user and be a joint experience. Hamill et al. (2008), in their qualitative study of service user's experiences of receiving the reformulation letter, found that the main theme from interviews indicated the use of the RL in connection (to themselves, to the therapist, to the therapeutic processes and to others). If the service user does not turn up for their planned RL session, the letter should be retained until you meet again, and never sent via email or post for them to read for the first time alone.

There can be differing ways of sharing a reformulation, based upon the service user's differing needs. We explore these within the next section below. In general, when working face to face with the service user, it can be useful to have two printed copies of the letter to hand, one to give to the service user in the room, and one for yourself. The following is a useful example of the narrative used to introduce the service user to the process:

> *I am going to give you a copy of your reformulation letter. I will read it aloud to you, and you can either just listen or follow along with me. It's helpful if you don't skip ahead, and just stay with me, so we can experience the letter together. If you feel you need me to stop at any time, just let me know and we can take a break. We will have time together at the end of the letter to discuss it in more detail. Do you have any questions?*

Reading the letter to the service user whilst they follow is a standard structure in CAT. This can be a skill in itself for the therapist, as they have to feel confident in reading aloud, not rushing the letter and also keeping an eye on the service user's reaction to the letter whilst hearing it. If you notice the service user is upset, you may want to pause, take a moment's silence, and then check in to see how they are and if they would like a break or for you to continue. At the end of reading the letter, it is often useful to give space to the service user. In doing so, you are allowing them to have the first word or are observing how they respond to the letter once it has been read. This is often telling information and together you can quickly be pulled onto the map as emotions may be running high. For example: does the service user fold the paper up and tuck it away in their handbag (in a bid to escape the emotion and push it to the back of their mind?), or do they hold the paper tightly, re-reading paragraphs (not wanting it to stop)? Such reactions can be helpful to observe and take a mental note of, as you may come back to them later at a time that feels comfortable, to think about in relation to the service user's map. As with all periods in therapy, sit for as long as the silence feels comfortable, if the service user remains quiet and you are unsure of their reaction, it may be worth using an open-ended question such as: 'How are you feeling?' or 'Do you have any thoughts?'

The remaining time in the session can then be spent discussing the service user's response to the letter, any particular areas that resonate with them, any inaccuracies or parts they disagree with and how they feel about the identified target problem procedures. This may develop further into thinking together about reciprocal roles and problematic patterns.

Different ways of sharing a letter

The previous section provides a generic structure to sharing the reformulation letter with the service user. This does not mean, however, that this is the only way it 'should' or 'could' be done. Along with the therapist's personal style, there can also be alternate and creative ways of sharing the letter differently. The format of sharing the letter can be altered, depending upon service user need, perceived benefits to them, or even when ways of working are different to usual (e.g., increased online working during and following the pandemic).

At times, some CAT practitioners feel the value of writing the letter collaboratively in therapy, particularly if the service user is worried about its contents, or if there is a fear that the 'presentation' of its contents may be too overwhelming or re-traumatising for the service user. In co-constructing the letter, the service user can then take ownership of what is written, and the contents can be discussed in more detail, aiming to further strengthen the therapeutic relationship. This might be particularly useful for people who have experienced feeling 'done to' or powerless in relation to others in the past. In adopting this approach, it is important to plan with the service user how you aim to deliver the letter, as if they are expecting you to share a prepared letter with them, and you have changed your mind/haven't written one due to lack of time, this can be detrimental for the service user, and they may feel disappointed in the change. If, however, you feel that collaboration in writing the letter will be beneficial for the service user, then this should be discussed and planned together in the prior session, so the service user feels comfortable and knows what to expect.

Being creative in the sharing of the RL can come as the therapist feels more skilled, and more confident in trying out alternate approaches to this stage of the therapy. Some practitioners may offer the service user an opportunity to respond in writing to the RL (a reciprocal approach to letter sharing is used in the goodbye letter, but generally not so often with the RL). This would be an open offer to the service user, with no consequences or repercussions, should they decide not to respond. Replying in letter format may allow the service user space to reflect and address their concerns or feelings in relation to the letter in an accessible and less daunting way.

The onset of the pandemic and the forced change to online working was a shock for practitioners, particularly in starting to provide therapy online. Over the last few years, we have become more skilled at this, and have experienced online therapy to be just as effective as in person. As a result, provision of online therapy has continued, even when restrictions have lifted, as it can be more convenient for both the therapist and the service user, due to reduced travel and no requirement for room bookings. We therefore need to consider clearly the most efficacious ways of delivering therapy online, so that collaboration is not compromised and the service user is able to engage just as easily through the virtual platform. The RL is one of the tools that has needed to be adapted through online sharing. Practitioners have found different ways of doing this, either through 'screen sharing', so that the service user can read the letter along with the therapist (whilst the therapist still watches for the service user's reaction, in the smaller screen), or through reading the letter aloud to the service user, whilst they listen, and then sharing it with them electronically, after the session has come to an end. Having delivered online therapy for almost two years now, Sarah has found that most service users ask for the letter to be read to them, rather than screen shared. This may be so they can maintain an easier view of the therapist, with fewer distractions in following the letter on the screen. In sharing this way, the process has not been unduly affected in any way.

Here, Andrew has provided his reformulation letter, from his contract of CAT. As mentioned in the opening chapter, both he and his therapist have provided consent for use of his CAT tools within the book. Names have been removed from the letter to maintain confidentiality of key people within Andrew's life. We would like to stress that this letter was written within the therapeutic relationship between Andrew and his therapist, and as such has meaning for the two of them together. The letter by no means should be taken as a definitive way of writing a reformulation letter, nor may it cover all of our guidance above in the 'how-to' of writing a letter but is presented here as an example and to give further detail to Andrew's therapeutic narrative.

Andrew's Reformulation Letter

This is a therapeutic letter not to be taken out of the context of CAT

Dear Andrew,
This letter is to summarise our discussions so far and to check we have a shared understanding of you and your difficulties. If you feel I have not got something quite right, then perhaps you can let me know so that we can amend it in a way that you feel better represents you.

You came to therapy because you were experiencing low mood, sleep disturbance and hurting yourself physically as a way of controlling your feelings. You had felt like this for some time, and you had begun to experience suicidal thoughts which you did not want to act on. Your previous counselling sessions had given you some knowledge about yourself, but you did not feel an emotional change at the end, and you were concerned about the impact this was having on those close to you.

We talked about what it was like growing up in your family, and how from the moment you were born you were given the message you are not capable of doing things 'right' and that those you most need and depend upon could be vulnerable and have the potential to leave you. This you may have sensed rather than 'known'. Your experiences of loss (your grandmother's death, your father's accident) were handled by you being 'excluded' from the family and left you bottling your anger and believing that your feelings are not important and that you are not capable of knowing what you need. I wonder if this exclusion felt a bit like an abandonment for you, as you were 'left' alone to manage yourself and hide your feelings, a bit like the schoolboy being wrongly accused and chastised by a teacher you had greatly admired and wanted to be close to. It must have felt a great letdown to be treated just like any other pupil and to learn that even people you admire can make mistakes. You have great memories of your Uncle coming to the rescue at times of critical need, and he is someone you really looked up to and admired and maybe you wanted to be like him, but by doing so setting yourself the impossible task of being an 'ideal', creating rules for yourself of how a man should be, thus striving to be who you thought you 'should be' rather than finding out who you really are? You had already learnt to 'hide' yourself and not trust your feelings so increasingly you felt a pressure to be who you thought you 'should be', becoming increasingly anxious about how others see you as you did not feel secure in yourself and learning to go along with others for fear of rocking the boat and being abandoned.

However, it seems when you are clear about what you really want, that you can commit to achieving it, such as holding your course to be a pattern cutter and your relationship with your wife and your friends. Work in the fashion business was not what you had imagined as there was the explicit expectation that your own needs would be unimportant, and you were drawn into striving to meet impossible standards for fear of critical attack and rejection by your demanding boss. Just as you reached the standard and had your patterns accepted, you were made redundant, so that rather than getting the admiration and recognition you had desired, you were left out on your own to fend for yourself. This you did, and perhaps driven by an underlying fear of failing, you set your own unachievable standards and took on too much, thus setting yourself up to fail and confirming your existing belief that you cannot trust yourself.

We have discussed how your difficulty with knowing who you are and accepting/trusting yourself underlies your difficulties now so that you feel as if you are always doing things to please others rather than knowing whether this is what you want. The goal of therapy is to help you know yourself a bit more and to connect with your feelings so that you can be more secure in yourself and trust yourself and your abilities.

The patterns that seem to keep your problems going are:

(1) Believing yourself to be no good, you set yourself impossible standards (perfection) in order to achieve admiration, recognition and approval. However, being impossible, these standards cannot be maintained, leaving you feeling dissatisfied, critical or exhausted.

(2) Fearing rejection and abandonment, you hide your feelings and needs for fear you will not be accepted. This leaves you feeling as if you are not being genuine and pulls you into criticising and dismissing yourself, thus hiding yourself further and leaving you feeling disconnected, alone and angry.

(3) Experiencing care as a means of control (and as if as a criticism that you cannot manage or others know best), you reject the care to manage by yourself but feel angry and resentful. You push yourself to achieve the impossible and set yourself up to fail, leaving you feeling alone, rejected, and worthless.

Over the remainder of the sessions, we will work on you becoming more aware of when these patterns are happening and how you may begin to change them. We will also need to be alert to when these patterns are happening between us, such as the ways you may hide yourself in therapy so that it could become an intellectual exercise and avoid the more painful feelings. We will also need to be mindful that as the sessions draw to an end that you may feel abandoned by me or disappointed when your expectations have not been met and disconnect from therapy and revert back to managing by yourself. How would we know if this were to happen? There is an opportunity to experience doing something different if you could flag up these things when you are aware of them happening and to learn to trust your feelings and be comfortable with showing yourself to others and risking the response. I look forward to the remaining work with you.

With Best Wishes,

[Therapist]

Andrew reflects here on what it is like to re-read his reformulation letter years later, and how this has helped to create a different relationship with himself.

Andrew says:

> *When I read my letter I just felt incredible sympathy, poor bugger feeling like that – I'm sat far away from it now, I'm far removed now – if I'd met me from then I'd just give me a hug and just tell me it's gonna be alright and sort of sit down and have a chat and say I know what you're going through and I know everybody's telling you you're gonna get through this and you really will, 'cos I'm you and I think CAT did an awful lot of doing that.*

Conclusion

It is hoped that this chapter is useful in aiding development of skills in writing and sharing a RL. The process of writing a RL is a time-consuming one, in terms of having the space to reflect, to write, to share in supervision and to make any amendments prior to sharing in therapy. Having space to do this within the therapist's day-to-day diary can be challenging and should be viewed with as much importance as the direct sessions themselves. Maintaining the collaborative stance in the sharing of the RL, through checking in with the service user's wellbeing and asking for their experience and thoughts on the RL, is key. The letter aims to deepen the service user's understanding of the self, how they relate to others, and what to expect throughout the course of therapy.

References

Hamill, M., Reid, M., & Reynolds, S. (2008). Letters in cognitive analytic therapy: The patients experience. *Psychotherapy Research*, 18(5), 573–583. https://doi.org/10.1080/10503300802074505

Newell, A., Garrihy, A. Morgan, K., Raymond, C., & Gamble, H. (2009). Receiving a CAT reformulation letter: What makes a good experience? *Reformulation*, Winter, 29.

Wilde McCormick, E. (2008). *Change for the Better*. Sage.

9 Mapping

Introduction

Within this chapter, the process of beginning to map is addressed, and how as a Cognitive Analytic Therapy (CAT) practitioner, we may begin to do this collaboratively with the service user. Once the service user has been introduced to the concepts of CAT, the therapist needs to consider how and when to start mapping. State mapping as a process in itself is considered, alongside how to use CAT concepts in the development of a Sequential Diagrammatic Reformulation (SDR). The SDR (CAT map) is the method of bringing together the notions of reciprocal roles and problematic procedures considered in the previous chapters, into an accessible, visual diagram for the service user. Additional aspects of the CAT map will be discussed, such as the use of the observing eye and healthy mapping.

When to state map?

As already mentioned, it is helpful to begin mapping with the service user as early as possible within therapy to capture themes which may be arising. State mapping is a useful way of starting to map with the service user, prior to beginning to develop a CAT map together. Ryle (2003) described a 'state' as being a distinct, contrasted way of being, feeling and acting. State mapping is not an essential requirement prior to CAT mapping, but it can be a useful way to start gathering your early understandings into diagrammatic forms, for example through identifying a key feeling or 'symptom' that your service user brings to discuss. They might also talk about states that feel starkly different from one another, for example, 'on a high' versus 'in a dark hole'. Not everyone will naturally think in a relational way or be able to access the detail of their linked thoughts and feelings to begin with, and CAT doesn't see this as a problem; it just means we start in a different place. As Potter (2004) suggests, we might think of states as "little knots of relational intelligence waiting to be loosened". Ryle (2003) introduced the States Description Procedure (SDP), a form developed for practitioners to use with service users who score above 28 on the

DOI: 10.4324/9781003308256-9

Personality Structure Questionnaire or identify a number of states within the last section of the psychotherapy file. The form allows for descriptions of the states which the service user is experiencing to be developed and for underlying reciprocal role procedures to be identified. The SDP is freely available to access to members of ACAT on their website.

In reflecting together about our own mapping skills, we recognise as CAT practitioners that we tend to map differently, with Sarah using state mapping more frequently with service users, whereas Jayne tends to reserve state mapping for more differentiated states which can occur for some service users. The reason for mentioning this at this point is to highlight that everyone maps differently. This isn't necessarily reassuring for a developing CAT practitioner, as often there can be a desire to ensure that it is done 'correctly'! However, an important piece of advice is to hold in mind that as long as the mapping is underpinned by CAT theory, is written within the service user's own words and makes sense to you and the service user, it will be 'good enough'.

Potter (2004) extended the self-states definition by suggesting that they are distinctive ways of feeling, thinking and relating which mediate *all* of our experiences. State mapping in itself can be useful as it can be the groundwork for more detailed mapping. It can be a way of orienting the service user to the process of drawing out key aspects of discussion on paper, giving them dialogical intensity (Potter, 2004). State mapping can begin through identifying key themes that have come up for you and the service user so far in the initial sessions. Sometimes the states are very distinct (e.g., the outgoing self versus the intimidated self). At other times, state mapping can be a way of noting down different key emotions which the service user frequently experiences and exploring them in more detail (e.g., criticised, cut off, isolated). Through starting with a blank piece of paper, these feelings or states can be randomly placed on the sheet (see Figure 9.1).

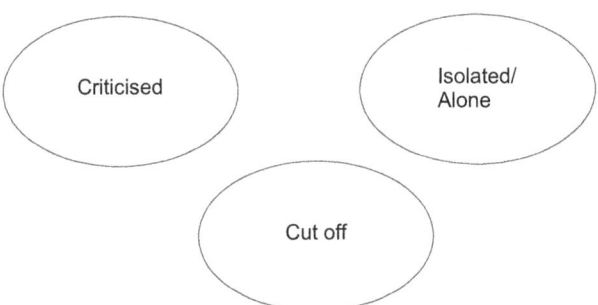

Figure 9.1 Early state mapping.

The therapist can then follow up the feelings with questions to explore further the personal meanings they have for the service user. Questions can include:

What does it feel like when you are in this place?

Can you describe it to me further?

Can you give me an example of a time when you have found yourself in this position?

This reminds me of when we discussed this experience … within the assessment. Is that true?

What do you think about yourself and/or others when you are in this place?

What makes this other place here feel so different?

What might have happened to lead you to feel this way?

As you are asking questions, you can note key words or phrases on the paper which relate to each individual state. Often, states are drawn with circles around them to distinguish them from one another. States are understood to refer more directly to the real subjective experience. They can be fleeting or chronically endured (e.g., the service user becomes stuck in them, unsure of how to escape).

There can be times through state mapping when the service user may begin to identify the problematic patterns they encounter. For example: if discussing a criticised state, the service user may allude to having to make sure they 'get it right the next time' (and the possibility of a perfectionist trap). It is worth exploring this further with the service user through asking more about what happens when they aim to 'get it right'. At this point, you are not actively mapping the procedure (this will come later in CAT mapping), but you can use these patterns to begin linking states together (see Figure 9.2). In doing so, you are working at the service user's own pace, and beginning to increase their recognition of potential patterns, before you map this more formally.

The formation of an early state map sets the scene for collaboration. The process of sitting side by side and seeing the creation of a map from a blank piece of paper can be very powerful. This shared understanding and communication sets a precedent for the service user feeling 'heard' and creates a space between the service user and therapist which acknowledges joint understanding. State mapping can also lead into the process of developing a CAT map more easily and suggests to the service user that the foundation of knowledge is there, but there is growth and expansion in considering procedurally what is going on for the service user.

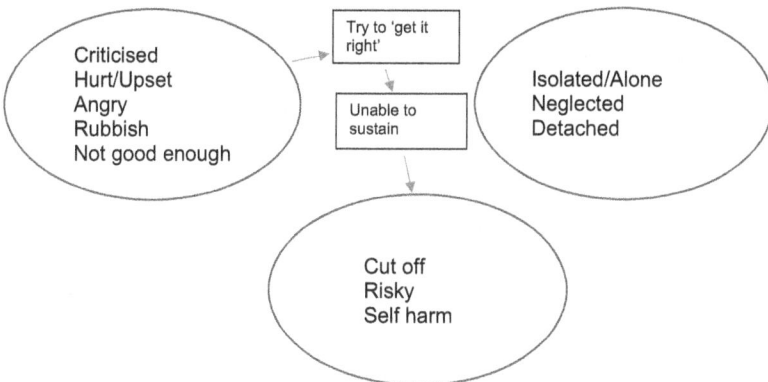

Figure 9.2 Developing a state map.

How do I start to map?

The 'when' and 'how' of beginning to map are probably frustratingly subjective; whilst traditionally the CAT model may have guided the trainee therapist to begin mapping after the reformulation letter (session 5 onwards); there has been, over time, an increasing recognition that we might start to map from our very first session. Here we will consider some key factors in deciding how and when to start mapping, in the hope that this will guide you through what can feel like a mysterious process to the beginning therapist.

All CAT practitioners will have different 'ways in' to start the CAT map. The two most important questions to ask yourself whenever you start to map are (1) Is the service user ready to see this on paper? and (2) Does this make sense to us both? A golden rule is to *use the service user's own words*. We can't really emphasise this enough. A danger is that we over-rely, in our uncertainty, on 'off the shelf' lists of common reciprocal roles when beginning to develop a map. It might be true that there are a finite number of possible reciprocal roles that we as human beings can inhabit (that's a debate for another day) – but there are likely to be infinite ways that we experience, describe and think about these ways of relating.

So, how might we start to map? It is important to try to listen to what a service user is telling you (both verbally and non-verbally) with your 'CAT ears'. So – listen not just for what they seem to be saying about themselves and others but how you are feeling in relation to them in the room. Be careful to be curious and tentative (particularly with the second part) and to listen for common themes. When you think you have a sense of something important, suggest to the service user that you would like to write down what has just been said, capturing it in a diagrammatic way, that makes sense to both of you. Let's use a theoretical example to help think this through.

Perhaps the new service user has come to their first therapy session and started to tell you that they often feel *taken advantage of* by others, that they *struggle to say no* and end up *doing too much*, leaving them feeling *exhausted* by the end of the day. If this seems to be a key or recurring theme you could tentatively map out the words *'taken advantage of'* on a piece of paper. As you're writing this down, you might say something like:

> *It sounds as though you can often be in this place (pointing to the paper) where you can feel as though others are taking advantage of you. Is that right?.*

If they indicate that this is correct (and their non-verbal communication is saying the same thing), you could also extend upon this in one of a few different ways. First, though, note that the words written down (out of the ones above in italics) are the ones that most closely indicate a pain-inducing *relational dynamic* of some sort (at a basic level in this example, something that is going on between two people) – however, all of the other parts of this narrative are key components of this role and related behavioural procedure too (i.e., 'doing too much' and 'feeling exhausted'); you will come to these a little later in mapping.

Once *'taken advantage of'* is mapped out on the piece of paper, there are a couple of different paths you could go down next. You may choose to try and map out the 'other end' of the role (*So, when you feel taken advantage of, what does it seem that other people are doing in relation to you?*) – the service user may answer 'using me' or 'taking advantage'? You could then draw this out as two ends of a role as depicted in Figure 9.3.

Alternately, you could clarify how they feel when they experience others as taking advantage of them. They might tell you they feel 'hurt', 'angry' or 'sad', and these feelings could be added to the bottom end of the role, perhaps in brackets or just underneath the box. Lastly, you might ask about what they *do* when they feel taken advantage of (alongside all the emotions, physical sensations, thoughts, urges and memories that are attached to this place).

Here, you are trying to get an idea of the procedure that is associated with this role. Procedures are usually our best attempts to move away from, mitigate or deal with a place that is painful or potentially painful. If the service user struggles to say no or act assertively, their feelings of hurt and anger due to being taken advantage of may build up. Eventually, they may find themselves

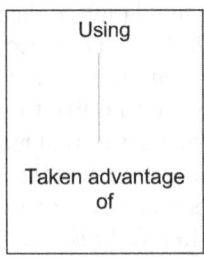

Figure 9.3 Development of a reciprocal role.

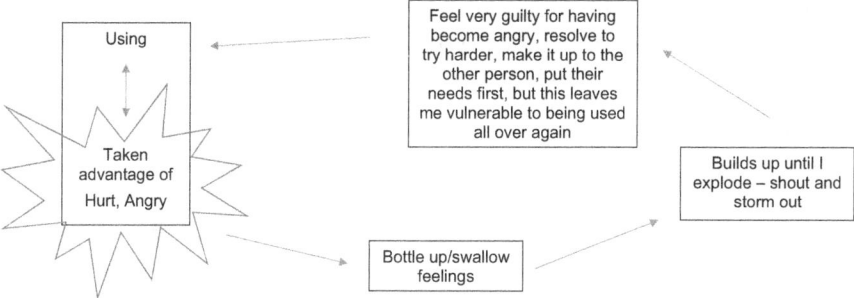

Figure 9.4 Development of a map.

having an angry outburst, feeling subsequently guilty and resolving that they should do more for the other person to make up for this. This unfortunately leaves them at risk of being taken advantage of all over again. Figure 9.4 shows the development of an early map, with the reciprocal role and initial problematic pattern evident.

On the other hand, if the service user is bringing a very specific example of something that happened this week, or earlier today, an example that is still 'hot', emotionally speaking, you may choose to map this out with them. There is no 'right' way to do this (although those of you who are familiar with behavioural chain analysis might find this a helpful comparison) other than to use the service user's own descriptions whilst you try to draw out a sequence of associated events, interpretations, thoughts, feelings and actions. This is another (equally valid) 'way in' to start mapping. Although your eventual aim is to develop a more general map, which is a higher-level shorthand for lots of similar examples, mapping a specific event is a great way to help the service user slow down and make sense of a procedure and also helps you as a therapist to start to build a more detailed sense of their internal world.

Whenever and however you start to map, you will be alert to how the service user is relating to the process itself. As mentioned earlier, the most crucial point here is that mapping should be a collaborative endeavour; maps emerge from dialogue and from shared sense making; they should be constructed jointly with the service user and never drawn up independently by the therapist outside of sessions and presented to the service user as a 'done deal' (Potter, 2010).

Developing a CAT map

As we have mentioned already, the process of developing a CAT map varies from therapist to therapist. Moving to the process of developing a CAT map is seen as increasing the higher level self/other reflection, through identifying reciprocal roles and problematic patterns (Potter, 2004). Whereas the states identified are more introspective (e.g., I am lonely, I am alone), the CAT map begins to explore the reciprocal nature of relationships. It can often feel different to move from state map to start CAT mapping; using the state map as the foundation, however, allows for the CAT map to be built upon it (e.g., develop the thinking further). Using the psychotherapy file at this point can help too with mapping as the service user and therapist can begin to draw together those frequently experienced procedures (which should align with key feelings identified in the state map).

Jefferis (2021) indicated a 'torchlight' model of working together on therapy maps, where the CAT concepts, therapist and service user come together through collaboration, placing focus on building the therapeutic relationship and shared understanding of the main reciprocal roles and problematic patterns. In CAT, the map is central to the therapy, and can begin only when there is trust and a 'good enough' relationship. The dialogue between the service user and therapist in jointly working on developing a map promotes a shared language and mutual effort.

Linking it all up – using BAPARF

The BAPARF acronym (as introduced in Chapter 5) can be a useful conceptual tool when beginning to construct CAT maps – it stands for 'Belief, Aim, Plan, Action, Result, Feedback' and applies most obviously to the mapping of circular 'trap'-based patterns but can be a useful tool to help you think more generally about how a service user 'moves around' their map. Once you've started to map out examples or common themes and begin adding key words, roles and procedures to your map(s), you will naturally start to think about how all of these 'part maps' join together into a coherent whole. From the assessment sessions, the completion of the psychotherapy file, state map and the reformulation letter, you should now have a good enough idea of the most important symptoms, feelings, behavioural patterns and ways of relating for the service user. You will also likely have an idea of their 'core pain' – in other words, the most painful place for them to occupy, often linked to key early experiences, which they will try to avoid at all costs.

You can ask the BAPARF questions from any place on the map and see where it takes you. For example, if we go back to the service user above, who often felt taken advantage of by others – we might have recognised that they are terrified of feeling 'not good enough' or being criticised. This place could represent their 'core pain'. We might use the BAPARF framework to try to understand what procedures arise from the 'not good enough' role and how this links up with other places on their map.

Belief – "I'm no good"
Aim – "to avoid criticism"
Plan – "strive hard to be good"
Action – "always say yes"
Result – "I initially avoid criticism and conflict but eventually burn myself out, miss deadlines and let others down"
Feedback – "I'm no good and must try harder"

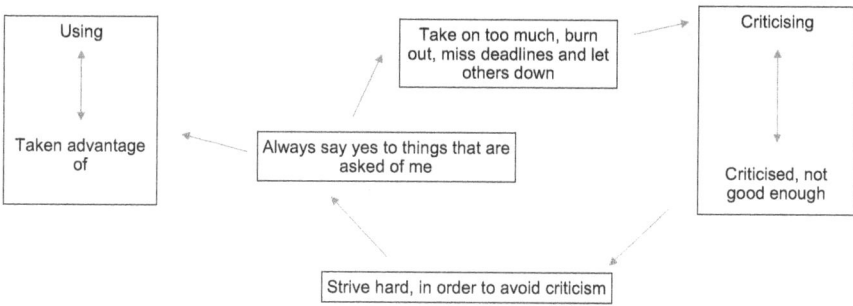

Figure 9.5 Map with two procedures.

From the above information we can see how this procedure is both circular/ self-fulfilling – in that it takes the service user right back to the feared place they started from, but also how it might link up with the role we already have mapped out – the "using to taken advantage of" role. We might then draw out two different possible procedures from the bottom of the 'not good enough' role: one (the above BAPARF) which takes them around in a circle and right back to the same place and another, which shoots off from the 'always say yes' action up to the 'using to taking advantage of' reciprocal role, because it is understandable to start to feel taken advantage of if we always say yes to everything, even when we don't want to or can't manage to do it. Figure 9.5 gives the diagrammatic version of this map, showing how the procedures link to the reciprocal roles.

You might remember that another possible outcome for the service user was an angry outburst following building resentment over being taken advantage of – this could easily be an alternative 'result' in the above BAPARF, and we might then map these two possibilities out as a 'dilemma' – that is, 'either I put up and shut up *or* I angrily explode' – as though these are the only possible two options when feeling aggrieved and taken advantage of. The way in which we might map this out is depicted in Figure 9.6.

We can then see how this false choice, or dilemma, can lead to the service user becoming so angry that they explode and verbally attack the other in 'an angrily attacking to hurt' reciprocal role in which they can at times occupy the pain-inducing role. The subsequent feelings of guilt and self-criticism they may experience after such an event would no doubt take them back into the 'not good enough' place at the bottom of their map, and so, in Figure 9.7 we can see how several different parts of the map are related to one another and can be viewed as a coherent 'whole'.

You will notice how the core pain or 'dreaded place' is at the bottom of the map as this usually seems to make intuitive sense. We will often draw out the places people are ideally trying to get to at the top of the map, with the ways they try to get there somewhere in the middle. This is more obvious on some maps than others; for the existing service user example, their map may be more focussed upon the need to avoid the place at the bottom, and the consequences

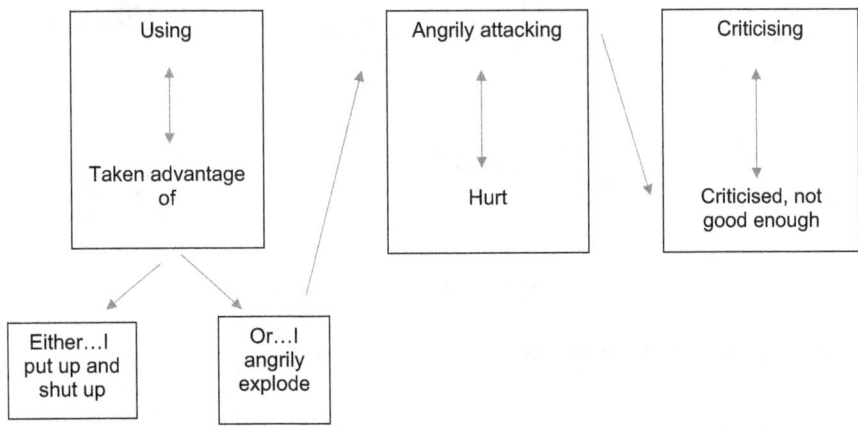

Figure 9.6 Developing map.

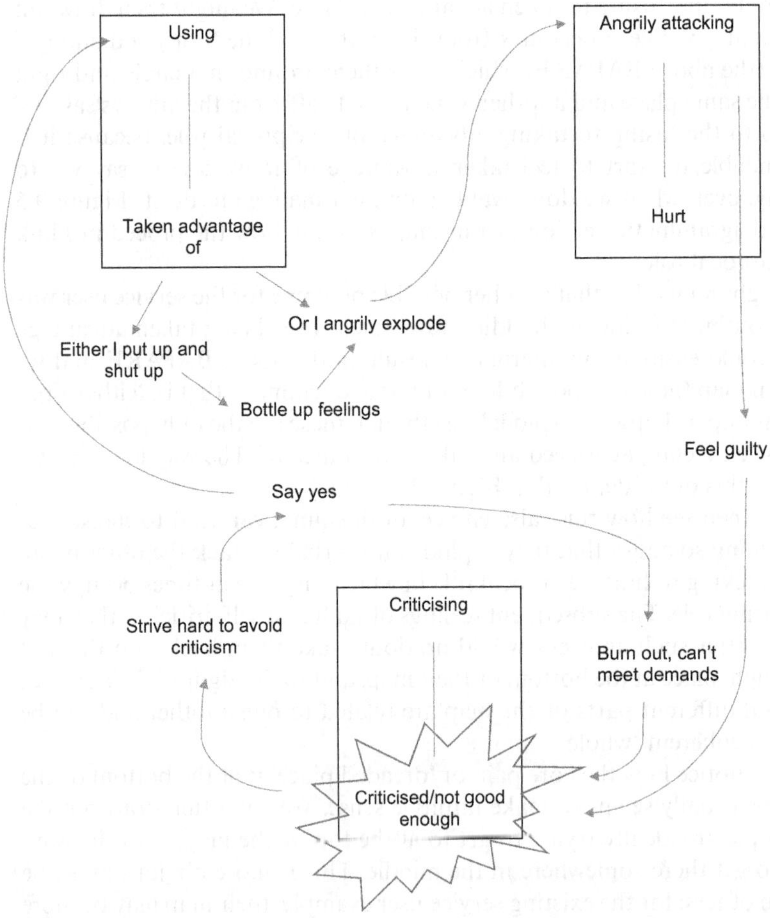

Figure 9.7 A CAT map.

that result from the ways they try to do this. However, for others there may be a stronger sense of a desired or 'wished for' place that they strive to occupy, and the resultant difficulties that can occur when this falters. As Ryle (1975) explained, knowing one end of a reciprocal role not only gives us an idea of its partner, but also suggests to us the contrasting, or *absent*, pair of roles. A reciprocal role of 'neglecting-to-neglected' naturally implies knowledge of 'caring-to-cared-for'; for some, the experience of the latter may have been present but inconsistent; for others, it may have been almost entirely absent and experienced only in the idealised realms of imagination.

Key features

Whilst mapping is not a 'one size fits all approach' and every map should be person-centred, using the service user's language to form reciprocal roles and problematic procedures, there are some key features that can be found on all maps (e.g., the observing eye).

Having a discussion with the service user about adding an 'observing eye' to the top of the map is important. The premise of the observing eye is to highlight the importance of recognition for the service user. It can be helpful to discuss with the service user how in the first instance, the observing eye may be yours as the therapist, and that you may notice problematic patterns with them. Through the process of the service user monitoring their patterns over the course of therapy, it is hoped that their own observing eye will become more developed.

As we map, we are ultimately beginning to increase the service user's observing eye, through recognition of key patterns. This can be difficult, as discussion may feel hard, at times exposing and painful. Shine and Westacott (2010) reported that whilst service users find the reformulation letter and the CAT map tangible objects to take away, they can be experienced as 'shocking' and 'exposing' due to the level of self-disclosure required. Here Andrew reflects upon his initial feelings on seeing the map start to take shape:

Andrew says:

> *The map, I'll be honest with you I was quite embarrassed by 'cos you're sat there going like 'oh yeah, I do do that, what do I do that for? Stupid!' – and I would say that to her and she's like 'right you're at that point now, you've just done that'… When someone writes it down, it's quite, you know a simplistic view, the way it goes to start off with and it can be quite obvious but 'cos you're in it, you're not seeing it and that fed into my insecurity 'cos I never thought I was particularly bright, so it's taken me 40 years or whatever to find this out, so right, I must be thick if it's taken me that long.*

The service user's reaction to the map is bound to be idiosyncratic; for Andrew, who does have a 'criticising-to-criticised' reciprocal role, there will always be the risk of viewing the very construction of the map through this lens. If the person you are working with can verbalise their thoughts and feelings in relation to the map, these can be made sense of and explored or challenged in the moment. It is perhaps worth reminding service users that we all have a 'map' and that even for those of us who are in the business of self-reflection, it's impossible to hold it in mind all the time. When you're in it, it can be almost impossible to see it, and it is therefore no surprise that others might be able to see it more clearly than us, at least to begin with. This speaks to that handing over of the observing eye that we spoke of above and is illustrated by how Andrew felt about his map later on in therapy:

Andrew says:

> *What I found interesting as well was as the map progressed, you know, it started that she would say 'you're at that point', you know I would say something and then, 'ooh, I'm at that point', it was starting to finally sink in that, right, OK I can spot where I am now and yeah I felt that was really sort of powerful as well it's almost like I can programme me sat-nav, I know which way this is going now you know I know roughly where I want to be and I know which are the bad streets so, whereas before I'd have to have someone telling me that.*

In addition to this, it is always important to remind the service user that the map is there to identify some of their main struggles, and thus the focus can feel challenging. As a result, the recognition that the service user too has a number of positive qualities that aren't yet mapped is also beneficial. Therapists tend to do this by adding a statement to the top of the map such as 'this is not all of me', or 'this is only part of me', to remind the service user that the difficult patterns don't define the whole of them.

Historically, to identify the service user's strengths and positive resources, a 'healthy island' was added to the map (usually depicted with a palm tree in the corner of the page, and words to represent the service user's protective factors).

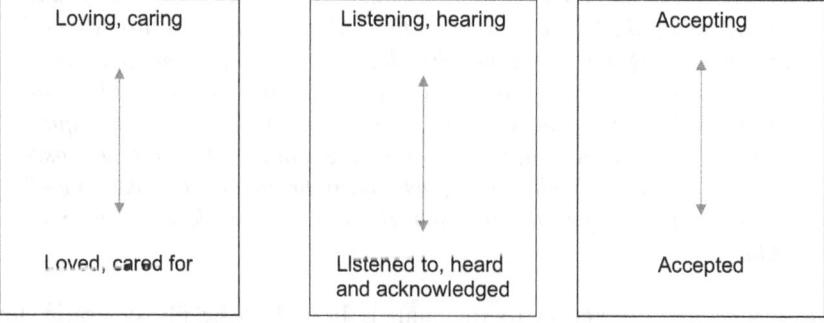

Figure 9.8 Healthy map.

The use of the healthy island has over time changed, with it being challenged as not representing enough of the service user's strengths on the map and visually appearing overshadowed by their difficulties. As a result, therapists now tend to collaborate with the service user to draw a 'healthy map' in its own right, using the concept of reciprocal roles and procedural patterns to identify healthy relationships (see Figure 9.8).

Below both Andrew and Karen have kindly shared copies of their CAT maps to show how their own experiences were depicted during therapy in diagrammatic forms (see Figure 9.9 for Andrew's map and Figure 9.10 for Karen's map).

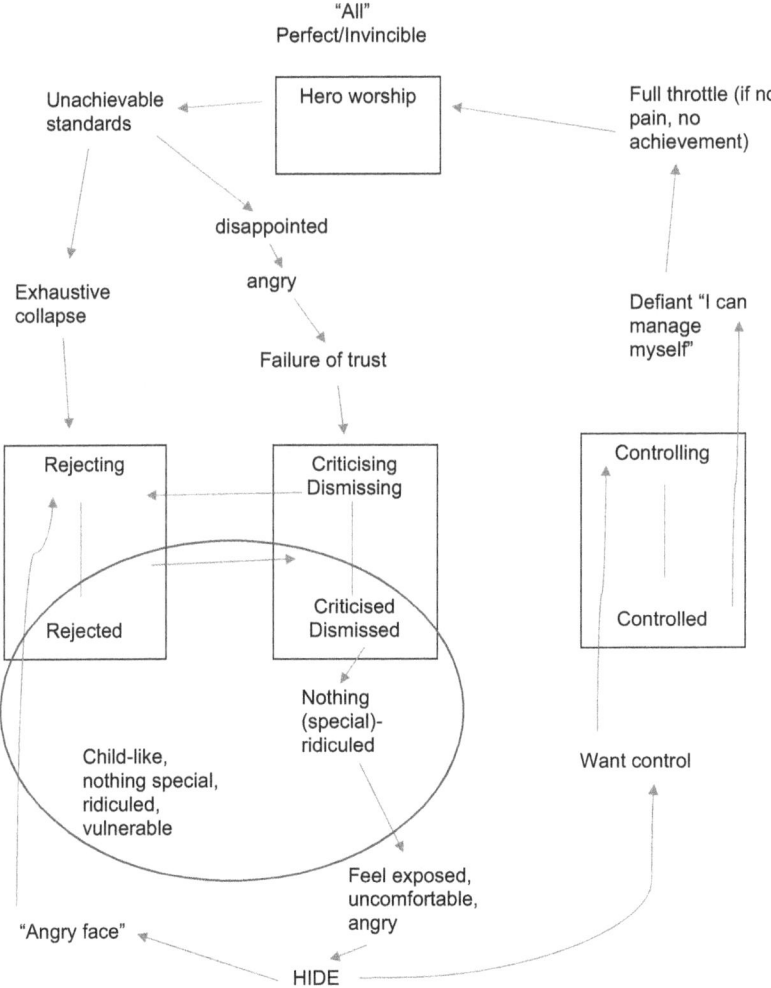

Figure 9.9 Andrew's map.

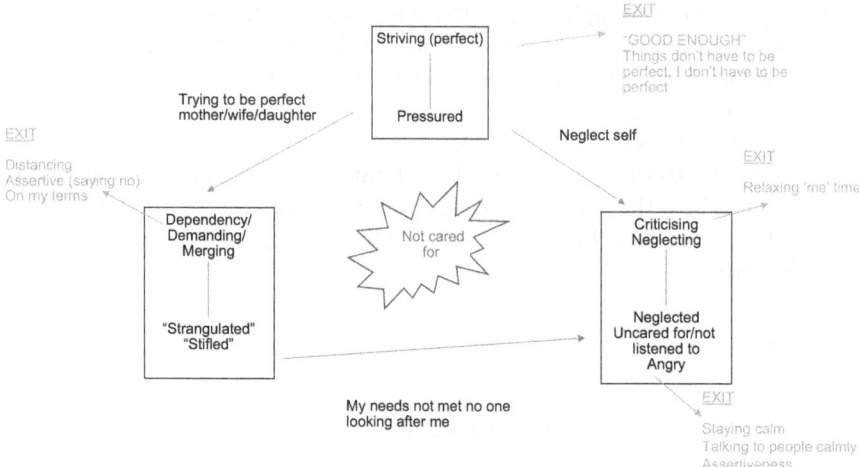

Target Problem: I find it difficult to deal with pressure from others. Unable to be assertive/too aggressive/fear of breakdown

Figure 9.10 Karen's map.

Conclusion

The CAT map is a central feature of CAT, which is developed collaboratively through the early sessions and remains visible and an active tool throughout the rest of the contract together. This chapter sets the scene as to how to begin mapping in the session, with the possibility of state mapping initially, followed by the integration of theory, evidence and practice in the development of an SDR. The key take-home messages for the therapist to remember in CAT mapping are the importance of the *collaborative* nature of the process, *using the service user's own words* on the map, *adding the observing eye* and reminding the service user that the map is *not a descriptor of all of them*. The map is always in draft form, and can be updated, added to or altered throughout the course of therapy. It is hoped that Chapter 11, which discusses the 'middle phase' of CAT, will emphasise further the importance of the map in the therapy room.

References

Jefferis, S., Fantarrow, Z., & Johnston, L. (2021). The torchlight model of mapping in cognitive analytic therapy (CAT) reformulation: A qualitative investigation. *Psychology and Psychotherapy: Theory, Research and Practice*, 94, 137–150. https://doi.org/10.1111/papt.12311

Potter, S. (2004). Untying the knots: Relational states of mind in Cognitive Analytic Therapy? *Reformulation*, Spring, 14–21.

Potter, S. (2010). Words with arrows: The benefits of mapping whilst talking. *Reformulation*, Summer, 37–45.

Ryle, A. (1975). Self-to-self, self-to-other: The world's shortest account of object relations theory. *New Psychiatry*, April, 12–13.

Ryle, A. (2003). The state description procedure. *Reformulation*, Autumn, 13–16.

Shine, L. & Westacott, M. (2010). Reformulation in cognitive analytic therapy: Effects on the working alliance and the client's perspective on change. *Psychology and Psychotherapy: Theory, Research and Practice*, 83, 161–177. https://doi.org/10.1348/1 47608309X471334

10 Monitoring

Introduction

Before we look at the middle phase of therapy, we explore in this chapter the process of monitoring within the recognition (the noticing of problematic patterns) phase of Cognitive Analytic Therapy. Whilst initially we tend to think of monitoring as occurring within the middle phase of CAT, it can begin to happen much sooner within the therapeutic relationship. This may be through service users' noticing patterns earlier within the contract, to more active tasks set with the service user to help them identify procedures whilst working through the mapping phase. As stated within previous chapters, often the different phases of CAT overlap, or merge, as aspects begin (e.g., monitoring), whilst others are being developed (e.g., the map). On the whole, monitoring marks the movement from reformulation to recognition; this represents a distinct shift in therapy, where the therapist and service user speak about naming patterns together, using the observing eye (initially the therapist's, with a view to increasing the ability of the service user).

Monitoring can occur in a number of ways, and here we will begin to explore each of these in more depth from classic to in-session recognition to personalised monitoring and the more creative methods.

Initial monitoring

Through mapping, the service user and therapist are jointly forming an understanding of the service user's difficulties. It is inherent within this process that the service user is beginning to recognise their own problematic patterns and reciprocal roles within their day-to-day life. We often hear the service user say, 'I know I do this'; however, they tend to then find it difficult to know what to do differently. There is a distinction between cognitively knowing you do something (in a generalised fashion) and the actual 'in the moment' recognition. Monitoring helps with the progression of recognition over time. The stages may include:

* Cognitively knowing – I can see how I avoid and bury my head in the sand when things get tough; it just happens.

DOI: 10.4324/9781003308256-10

- Suspended recognition – I felt dreadful yesterday; I couldn't face going into work, so I stayed at home in my pyjamas all day. It was only on the evening when I thought about it that I realised I was avoiding again.
- In the moment recognition – I could feel myself getting anxious about my exams next week, I was supposed to be studying but instead noticed I was procrastinating by doing jobs in the house. I stopped the jobs and sat down to study. I got so much done and felt better as a result.

There is little reported in the CAT literature about monitoring, despite it being a central feature in recognition. Generally, monitoring is tailored to the service user's own learning needs and ability to engage in work outside of the therapy. Initially, monitoring may take the form of 'looking out for' and recording in a diary when key reciprocal role procedures (RRPs) have been noticed (aiming to move the service user into a position of suspended recognition). As an initial map is formed together, the therapist may then introduce concepts of what we term more 'classical monitoring', using CAT monitoring sheets, which can be found for members of ACAT on their website.

Historically in CAT, monitoring has been paper-based. It often starts within the session and is advocated to be completed as a task outside of therapy, in the hope the service user will develop skills of 'in the moment' recognition. In doing so, the service user is also prompted to think about how they revised the problematic pattern, shifting the focus even further to exits and beginning to step out of the difficult procedure they have found themselves within.

Classic monitoring

Classic monitoring begins where the therapist uses the map as a tool to reflect back to the service user when they have 'noticed' a pattern occurring (either within the room or within the information shared by the service user of their day-to-day experiences over the course of the last week). Using the map between the service user and therapist can be helpful within the therapeutic relationship to suggest the possibility of a pattern occurring, in a non-threatening, enquiring way. The therapist may use questioning such as '*I wonder if …*', '*it seems like …*', '*I've just noticed …*'. Through such discourse, the therapist can aid the service user in thinking about their patterns and see how accessible the recognition phase is to them at this point in time. For example, the service user may agree with the 'wonderments' and take the reflection further, acknowledging other examples that the conversation has made them think of. On the other hand, the service user may disagree with the therapist's reflection, stating that this is not the case, and they did not see the pattern having occurred in this situation. The CAT literature speaks of "pushing where it moves" (Ryle, 1990), that is, if the service user is engaging in the recognition, the therapist can explore this further in order to deepen the understanding and reflections. If the service user is struggling to see the pattern, then the therapist may move the conversation on, in the understanding that if the reflection the therapist had made was accurate, the pattern will come up again at some point in the future.

As mentioned earlier, the growing ability of the service user to recognise patterns can come with a 'dip' in their mood in therapy, as they have a sense of 'knowing' without the ability to 'do something different'. Support within therapy at this time is key for the service user, to remind them that recognition without the revision phase can be hard, as you are able to observe what is taking you into the places of core pain without being able to stop this from happening. Encouraging the service user at this point to continue and reminding them that change will inevitably come are important.

There are two main monitoring sheets, which we refer to as the 'classic monitoring' in CAT, as these are long-standing, core tools which most practitioners use to help the service user to begin to identify their procedures. The tools are available to members of ACAT and accessible on their website, under the CAT tools section.

The first monitoring sheet is the Target Problem Procedure Rating Sheet. This tool is longitudinal in nature, using one sheet to span the whole of the therapy contract. The sheet incorporates a graphical figure, on which the service user is asked once a week to rate their ability to recognise and revise the identified TPP. The service user asterisks how skilled they feel to recognise the pattern (e.g., more skilled than usual, less skilled than usual, or the same as usual). The revision section of the graph takes the same format, asking the service user to depict on the graph how skilled they feel in revising the TPP (e.g., more skilled, less skilled or the same as usual). It is hoped that over the course of therapy, the service user becomes more skilled in being able to both recognise and revise the TPP, and thus, can see this improvement visually on the graph. The Target Problem Procedure Rating Sheet also allows for any exits identified outside of sessions to be recorded, and thus these can be discussed further as part of the next session. This rating sheet can be a quick and easy way for the service user to report back on their ability to recognise their TPP, instances in which the TPP has occurred and how they may have revised the pattern.

The second monitoring sheet is named CAT Weekly Rating Sheet for service users. This rating sheet differs from the TPP rating sheet in that it allows the service user to notice and in their own words record an explanation of up to three patterns each week. The service user is then guided to record on a Likert scale how able they were to notice the patterns (with 0 = not at all, 1 = after the event, 2 = during the pattern, 3 = early on). The ultimate aim of this scale is to enable the service user to think to a greater extent about the pattern, aiming for 'in the moment' recognition. In line with the movement towards revising the patterns, the service user is then asked over the last week how able they were to consider alternatives to each pattern (with 0 = not at all, 1 = thought about, 2 = talked about and 3 = tried something). Next the service user is asked to reflect on three problems over the last week and identify the extent to which each has troubled them (from 1 = not at all to 4 = extremely). Finally, the service user is prompted to reflect on the most positive aspect of the week. Whilst a visual representation of the service user's progress is not seen within this particular rating sheet, the service user is guided here to think more broadly about their problematic patterns and to spend more time considering their engagement within such patterns. An added benefit of this particular rating sheet is that in the final question, which asks the service user to identify a positive aspect of the week, it aims to move the service user away from their negative thinking and into recognition of healthier states and what has gone well.

Whilst this classical rating sheet is based on a weekly format, it can be adapted to meet the service user's needs. Andrew provides an example of his monitoring sheets, which he completed on a daily basis. The sheet shows his reflection on both the recognition and revision of patterns within a particular day (see Figure 10.1).

Daily Rating Sheet

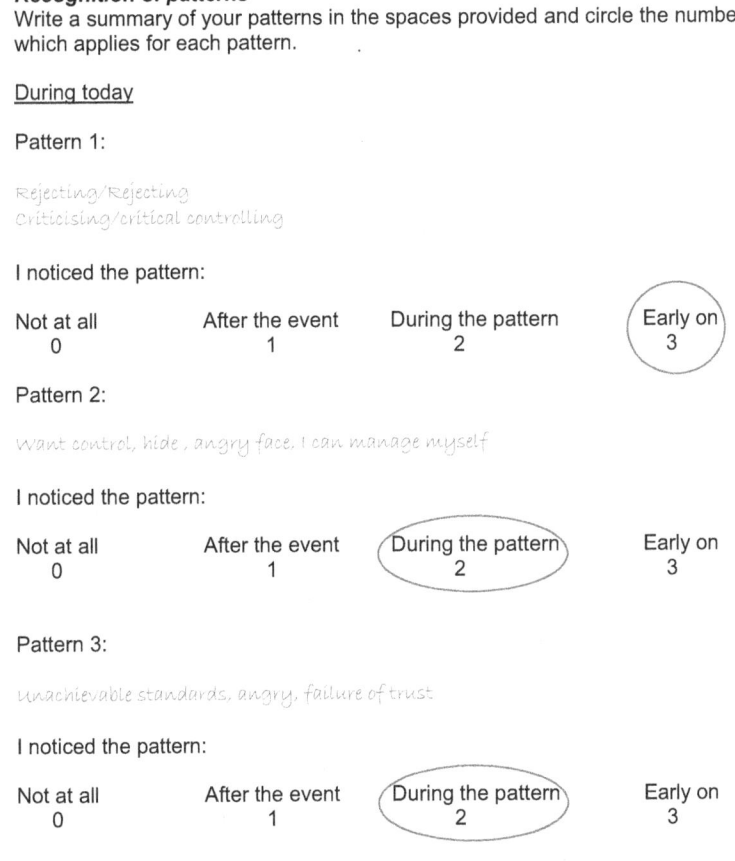

Recognition of patterns
Write a summary of your patterns in the spaces provided and circle the number which applies for each pattern.

<u>During today</u>

Pattern 1:

Rejecting/Rejecting
Criticising/critical controlling

I noticed the pattern:

Not at all   After the event   During the pattern   Early on
0   1   2   3

Pattern 2:

Want control, hide, angry face. I can manage myself

I noticed the pattern:

Not at all   After the event   During the pattern   Early on
0   1   2   3

Pattern 3:

unachievable standards, angry, failure of trust

I noticed the pattern:

Not at all   After the event   During the pattern   Early on
0   1   2   3

Figure 10.1 An example of Andrew's monitoring sheet.

(Continued)

Revision of patterns

<u>During today</u>

Pattern 1:

I considered alternatives:

Not at all	Thought About	Talked About	Tried Something
0	(1)	2	3

Pattern 2:

I considered alternatives:

Not at all	Thought About	Talked About	Tried Something
0	(1)	2	3

Pattern 3:

I considered alternatives:

Not at all	Thought About	Talked About	Tried Something
0	(1)	2	3

Problems

Please write a one/two word description of each problem in the space(s) provided and rate the extent to which each one has troubled you today.

	Not at all	A little bit	Moderately	Quite a bit	Extremely
Prob 1: *London visit*	0	1	2	(3)	4
Prob 2:	0	1	2	3	4
Prob 3:	0	1	2	3	4

Figure 10.1 (Continued)

On the whole, classical monitoring sheets are utilised routinely in CAT practice, yet there is little (or no!) evidence to report the efficacy of the use of these tools in therapy for service users. Harvey (1993) developed a TP and TPP rating sheet with a service user, which allows for recognition that there may be multiple target problem procedures feeding the target problem.

CAT tools are inherently based upon Cognitive Behavioural Therapy, with the therapist initiating an active phase within the therapy, whereby the service user is prompted to begin thinking about their own thoughts, feelings and behaviours and the impact these then have on their own difficulties. Such rating sheets can be used routinely by CAT practitioners, and their usage tends to be based on service user need alongside therapist preference for the tools. As authors writing this chapter, we identified we both have our own individual preferences, with Sarah more routinely using the TPP rating sheet whilst Jayne actively uses the individual pattern recognitions sheet! Often, however, such classical monitoring is not enough to engage the service user in their progress and period of change. In light of this, bespoke, personalised monitoring methods can be used to creatively facilitate recognition and revision.

Personalised monitoring

Involving the service user in developing their own monitoring sheets speaks to the principles of collaboration and person-centred care. We consider personalised monitoring to be just this, tailored to the service user's personal need. As we approach the middle phase of CAT, we find that drawing on other models to inform monitoring can also engage the service user in recognising their problematic procedures from an integrative approach. In particular, as mentioned above, this may incorporate the use of cognitive behavioural approaches to monitoring, such as thought records (if taking a more cognitive approach to challenging the service user's TPPs) or activity scheduling (for more behavioural approaches). It is often useful to think about adapting monitoring to tailor to the service user's needs. For example: activity scheduling can be used reactively for the service user to put into the schedule what they have done (and thus to look out for any patterns), or proactively (to plan tasks within the week), or as a red, amber, green (RAG) rating to monitor how much or little of tasks are completed (e.g. red – work; amber – housework; green- personal care).

Some service users may benefit from writing out their own procedural patterns in full (to highlight when they are occurring and what happened) by way of a journal or diary entry, whereas others may prefer to use a procedure tracking form (Kingerlee, 2004). The procedure tracking form is a standardised monitoring sheet developed on the underpinning premises of a CBT thought record but allows the service user to track their procedural sequence, holding in mind that affect, cognition, meaning and action are all linked (Ryle & Kerr, 2002). Kingerlee (2004) highlights that the procedure tracking form comprises five columns for the service user to complete which include: perception (what was the situation/what did you notice occurring?), appraisal (what sense did you make of the situation/what were you thinking?), enactment (what did you do/what reciprocal roles did you adopt?), evaluation (how did you feel after the event?) and confirmation/revision (what did you do differently/what could you do differently next time?). It is felt that taking time between sessions to actively self-reflect on each of these stages of a procedural sequence will positively impact the individual's psychological state and lead to a higher level of self-reflection (Kingerlee, 2004).

On the whole, it is helpful in monitoring to go with what works for the service user. Sometimes, personalisation of monitoring comes through joint ideas within the session. It is important to be flexible, to plan together and to put into place homework tasks which the service user feels happy to go away and do. Monitoring is not intended to be a burden; the aim is for it to feel manageable and understandable for the service user to complete.

Creative monitoring

As we move into a digital age, consideration has been made to moving CAT tools online. Easton et al. (2021) have begun to work on blending CAT with a digital support tool. Their aim is to develop a prototype digital mobile app, within which worksheets will be built in to aid the recognition phase of CAT. The app is being researched using a mixed-methods approach involving a user-centred design to see if it is feasible to use in practice. It is hoped that the app will allow easier access to CAT tools for the service user to utilise outside of therapy. Whilst such an advancement in technology will improve access for the service user, data protection and governance are an issue, to ensure that personal and sensitive information remains safe.

The barriers to monitoring

For the duration that CAT has been delivered, monitoring has taken place in paper format, with service users taking copies of their maps, letters and rating sheets home with them in a file. Such paper-based tools can be seen as inconvenient and impractical as they can be easily lost or forgotten and can create embarrassment for the service user if seen by others (Varela, 2016). Not having the required tools to hand throughout therapy can create a barrier for the service user and therapist in moving forward, particularly if rating sheets are not completed, left at home or misplaced.

Such occurrences can arise for any of us within life. We are only human and may forget to do something or to pick up a file we need as we are leaving the house. If you find that such incidents happen more frequently within therapy, it is important to begin to notice the pattern, to name it with the service user and to think openly as to why the homework or the rating sheets are not being returned. It may be that the service user is struggling for time to complete the monitoring at home, is worried that a family member will see the contents of the file or is finding it difficult to understand how to complete the monitoring sheets and what they mean. Having an open, non-critical conversation about the tools may help to exit from the pattern of non-completion or the barrier that is leading to this.

As mentioned above, developing digital means of storing and recording shared information in CAT between the therapist and service user may be a step towards eliminating some of these barriers which may occur (Varela, 2016).

Conclusion

Monitoring is an integral part of the recognition and revision phases of CAT. Its aim is to guide the service user outside of sessions in reflecting more deeply on their problematic procedures and considering alternate ways of doing something different. There are a number of different ways of facilitating monitoring for the service user, from utilising the CAT-specific monitoring sheets to adapting and personalising cognitive behavioural rating sheets to the service user's needs. We will no doubt see the development of further CAT-monitoring sheets in future years, particularly through more opportunity to complete rating sheets online or digitally through mobile apps.

References

Easton, K. et al. (2021). Blending Cognitive Analytic Therapy with a digital support tool: Mixed methods study involving a user centred design of a prototype app. *JMIR Mental Health*, 8(2), e20213. https://pubmed.ncbi.nlm.nih.gov/33522979/#:~:text=1%3B8(2)%3Ae20213.-,doi%3A%2010.2196/20213.,-Blending%20Cognitive%20Analytic

Harvey, L. (1993). On TP and TPP rating sheets. *Reformulation*, Autumn.

Kingerlee, R. (2004). The Procedure Tracking Form (PTF): A possible new tool for CAT. *Reformulation*, Summer, 25–27.

Ryle, A. (1990). *Cognitive Analytic Therapy: Active Participation in Change*. John Wiley and Sons.

Ryle, A. & Kerr, I. (2002). *Introducing Cognitive Analytic Therapy: Principles and Practice*. Wiley.

Varela, J. (2016). Developing a mobile application to support Cognitive Analytic Therapy. *Reformulation*, Winter, 37–38.

11　The middle phase

Introduction

As we have now explored the use of monitoring sheets within therapy, this leads us nicely into considering the 'middle phase' of CAT. CAT has been well known for its absence of literature surrounding the middle phase, and lack of direction as to what to do between sessions 5 and 15. The reason for this is predominantly due to its integrative nature and CAT practitioners working to engage the service user in a truly collaborative, person-centred approach to therapy. Therefore, it is difficult to name all that will go on in such sessions, as each therapy is tailored to the individual. Within this chapter, however, we aim to give you a general overview of the structure of the middle phase: we consider the overarching theories that underpin CAT, which we introduced you to in Chapter 3 (the cognitive/behavioural and analytic theories) and how these are used in the intervention phase, and we consider alternate approaches that can be drawn upon depending upon the service user's need. We also return to the concept of the healthy map and consider how this is used within the middle phase whilst also beginning to consider revision here, through the use of exits (which will be explored in more depth within the next chapter).

The routine of the sessions within the middle phase

When learning to practice CAT, it can be unnerving and anxiety-provoking for the therapist to face the expanse of the middle phase of therapy with little direction. There is no manualised approach to CAT, which makes it so unique, creative and exploratory. However, this can also be daunting, particularly as humans we like to know if we are doing something 'right' or 'wrong' when learning! Despite the lack of structure to the middle phase, there are some key considerations that you can hold in mind to provide yourself with a loose plan of how to organise sessions.

Firstly, in preparation for the session (ensuring the environment is conducive to therapy, e.g., noise level, lighting, seating arrangements, temperature, privacy ctc.), it is important to place the most up-to-date CAT map in the room where it can be seen, ready for the service user arriving. This can allow the service user

DOI: 10.4324/9781003308256-11

to feel held in mind, for the importance of the map to be implicitly acknowledged and for it to be easily accessible when needed throughout the session.

As mentioned previously, in welcoming the service user to the start of the session, it is always useful to 'count down' the number of sessions with them (e.g., *Today we are at session 7 out of 16*). Once again, this provides the service user with a structure, a boundary to the time you have together and acts as a reminder that the end of sessions will come. Counting of sessions also enables the therapist to highlight the mid-point of therapy (e.g., at session 8), and to provide space for the service user to be able to reflect upon what it feels like to reach halfway. Discussions can give an indication of how the service user is feeling in relation to their progress, their time in therapy and the inevitable ending. It allows for time to review the target problem and consider change in relation to this as well as to revisit aims and the likelihood of achieving them as the ending approaches. At the midway point, service users can tend to express a whole host of thoughts and feelings for example from 'feeling the therapy is going too quickly', 'not wanting the ending to come', 'feeling as though they are stuck or not progressing' or 'feeling as though they have a mountain to climb'. In sharing and naming these feelings together, the service user and therapist can openly acknowledge any difficulties and areas of change already experienced and identify continued areas to work upon.

CAT practitioners often begin the dialogue in session by recapping what may have happened in the last session, returning to any outstanding issues from the previous session that need addressing, and checking in with the service user on how the week has been for them. The generic opening of the conversation in hearing about the last week can allow the therapist to explore any areas of difficulty the service user has encountered (whilst holding the map in mind and any potential problematic procedures they may have been drawn into), any positive outcomes the service user identifies (which could be considered as exits on the map) and the service user's general emotional presentation at that point in time. It may be that the service user shares an example of an experience throughout the last week and the therapist aids the service user in a deeper understanding of the situation. For example:

Service user:	I was feeling generally good about myself until Friday. I missed the bus into work and as a result I was 45 minutes late. My boss was unhappy with me and said that if I am late to work anymore, I will be given a verbal warning.
CAT Practitioner:	How were you feeling as a result of this?
Service user:	I felt useless, I knew it was my fault I was late as I couldn't motivate myself to get out of bed. By the time I did, and I got myself ready and to the bus stop, I saw the bus pulling away.
CAT Practitioner:	So how did you manage at work?

Service user:	I apologised to my boss, but kept quiet for the rest of the day, I didn't want to talk to anyone and went to lunch on my own. I felt so alone.
CAT Practitioner:	If we have a look at your map together, do you think you can spot where you might have been on this occasion?
Service user:	I felt blamed by my boss for being late, and so I withdrew from the situation, leading me to feel all the more alone. I didn't realise that at the time, but it made me feel so low.

It is often useful to leave ten minutes or so towards the end of the session to prepare the service user that it is drawing to a close, to share any final reflections on the session, set tasks for the next week to be completed outside of sessions and to answer any queries in regard to this. Saying goodbye at the end of each session can mirror separation anxieties which may be felt in the wider ending of the therapy contract. The service user may experience feelings of rejection or abandonment (if these emotions are central to the map) in relation to you or may pull you to want to extend the session or find it difficult to say goodbye. There can be times in which the service user ends the session with a disclosure or a key piece of information (also known as a "doorknob comment", Koons, 2016), which is often understood in the literature as being due to finding it too difficult to share in the session, wanting to offload the pain of the experience, wanting you to be the perfect therapist or wanting to keep you longer. Such 'foot in the door' experiences can be difficult to manage as a therapist and can lead to you being pulled to 'join the dance' with the service user. Maintaining boundaries of session timings is always important, as it provides the service user with a secure base from which they can return to their 'outside world' and allows the service user to feel a sense of consistency with regards to what to expect in the structure of the sessions. If a threat to maintaining the boundaries occurs for any of the reasons suggested above, it is important to hold what the service user is bringing (assess risk and manage accordingly), acknowledge its significance and that you will return to it at the start of the following session (the vital aspect of this being that you do raise it at the start of the next session!).

Towards the end of the session, always offer the service user an up-to-date copy of their map, exits and monitoring sheets (which can be photocopied and provided to the service user at the end of the session if face to face or securely sent to the service user via email if online). Karen explains some of her memories of the middle phase of therapy and the interventions used by the therapist.

Karen says:

I just remembered her doing the drawings, but obviously the effect it had was massive. I couldn't talk about my childhood without crying all the time and that's where I was up to, and I knew I had to go back and examine things and even at the point where it was really affecting me. When she said about talking to my mam about why I was left as a young child with the neighbour and things like that. And she said, 'go home, write a letter and get all those feelings out'. And then I thought, no, I'm gonna go talk to my mam about it and she couldn't believe it when I went back and she said, 'did you write the letter then?' And I said, 'no, I went and talked to mam and I'm so glad I did as she accepted that things weren't right and that things shouldn't have happened'. And we massively built coverage and thank God we did because little did I know shortly down the line she was gonna get dementia but that helped me not to hold any resentment and kind of like clear the air so it massively did; it was just the right time for me as well.

The C in CAT

Within the broader framework of the CAT model there are many interventions that can be drawn upon within the middle, or active, phase of therapy. As we have previously discussed, the influence of cognitive therapy upon CAT is perhaps most obvious at a 'whole model' level in its structured, collaborative, problem-focussed nature. At the level of problem conceptualisation and intervention there are of course also many parallels. If early recognition and monitoring has been successful, by this point in therapy we will have an early draft or drafts of the map and some week-to-week examples of times when patterns have emerged inside or outside of therapy. Key cognitive and behavioural interventions at this stage may include thought challenging, behavioural experiments and activation, bodily relaxation techniques and graded exposure. These will all be situated within and emerge from the broader CAT (re)formulation, rather than being applied in a 'scattergun' type approach but may be particularly relevant when exploring TPPs using the BAPARF (belief, aim, plan, action, response, feedback) sequence. For example, in recognising the belief that underpins a sequence of action (e.g., 'I must keep my feelings bottled up' or 'people will find me boring' or 'I'm no good at this'), we are afforded an opportunity to step back from and examine this thought in more detail. Whilst more traditional methods of cognitive restructuring (i.e., the downward arrow technique, weighing the evidence for and against a negative thought) may be sufficiently helpful to some, others will benefit instead from considering the usefulness or helpfulness of the thought itself. Third wave cognitive approaches (e.g., Acceptance and Commitment Therapy [ACT], Mindfulness Based Cognitive Therapy [MBCT]) may encourage a more explicit 'cognitive defusion' or 'stepping back from' the thought, rather than engaging in an evaluation of its 'truth'. All these interventions may take place at the level of core belief, intermediate assumption or negative automatic thought, depending upon the specificity of the example being mapped. Similarly, at the 'aim' and 'plan' level of the procedure, it may be possible to step back from these potential 'rules for living' and explore the validity of the assumptions made therein.

Following the imaginary service user who we mapped in Chapter 9, we can conceptualise examples of potential cognitive interventions that may be useful for them. Remember that to escape from the position of feeling 'not good enough' they strived hard to avoid criticism and always said yes to things that were asked of them. Imagine that a rule for living underlying this procedure was something like 'if I'm not perfect, then I will be criticised by others (which will prove to me that I am not good enough)' – it may be possible to step back from and examine the usefulness of this rule or even challenge the core belief underlying it (i.e., 'I'm not good enough') for example by using a continuum method (a process used to challenge unhelpful beliefs) to help establish a more realistic sense of self.

Similarly, the behavioural elements of CBT can be brought to the table in working upon the 'Action, Response and Feedback' elements of the procedure. This might be direct behavioural experimentation (for example, the service user making a conscious planned alteration to one of their usual 'safety behaviours' and assessing the outcome) or an informal 'graded' exposure to previously feared situations, thereby tackling the negative consequences of avoidance. Following our imaginary service user, we may for example plan with them a behavioural experiment to test out the assumption 'If I am not perfect, then I will be criticised by others'. As with all CBT-based interventions, it is crucial that the service user has a good understanding of the rationale for the methods of intervention used. We propose that CAT would perhaps add to this a focus upon the importance of the service user understanding the relational *origins* of the procedures as a way of surviving prior adversity.

The A in CAT

In true 'analytic' style, the A in CAT underpins the approach from a deeper relational and collaborative perspective. Relationships underpin all our interactions as humans, whether they be in relation to the self or to others. The therapeutic relationship offers the service user opportunity to experience alternate patterns to what they may have encountered in the past (through the therapist actively aiming not to collude or reciprocate problematic procedures). As a result, an alternative relationship can be modelled and can unconsciously aid vicarious learning. On the whole, we consider the analytic perspective in CAT as relating to reciprocal roles, the concepts of which can be recognised and discussed within the therapy. Bennett (1995) identified that service user's maladaptive and interpersonal patterns will emerge in the relationship with the therapist and are therefore a useful source of information. The therapist will use the therapeutic relationship and the dialogue about relationships outside of therapy to make tentative interpretations and to begin to identify reciprocal roles with the service user. This can happen on a session-by-session basis. There does not need to be a rupture within the relationship to talk about relational patterns, although therapeutic ruptures in themselves (if considered in relation to the map) can aid change (see Chapter 15 for a further consideration of therapeutic ruptures).

Bennett (1995) identified a model for enactment resolution in the therapeutic space, suggesting guidance that can be helpful for beginner therapists, as often challenges between the therapist and service user can be anxiety-provoking and difficult to manage for both. Such stages of enactment resolution include:

1. *acknowledgement of an in-session experience (name with the service user what you have noticed between the two of you and how it would be helpful to consider it further, in the here and now)*
2. *exploration (spend time discussing what happened between the two of you, and how you both felt as a result)*
3. *link it to the SDR (can the service user notice where the two of you might have been on the map and identify any reciprocal role enactments?)*
4. *explanation (think together about where the reciprocal role procedure came from and its history)*
5. *negotiations of understandings and disagreements (How could the situation have been different? Is there a way that you could have stepped out of the pattern together?)*
6. *coming to a consensus (How will you resolve the situation and step out of the RRP together?)*

Analytic theory considers the use of transference and countertransference (see Chapter 3 for a reminder of these concepts), which can also be useful within the exploration of what may happen between service user and therapist within the room. As we have stressed already, the formation of the working alliance early in therapy can aid shared understanding and, in the event of transference and countertransference, can allow for work to be continued. King (2005) highlighted that transference entails a misperception or misinterpretation of the therapist whether negative or positive, where countertransference refers to the feeling that a therapist experiences towards the service user. Ryle and Kerr (2020) referred to two types of countertransference that the therapist needs to bear in mind: their personal countertransference (what they as a therapist bring to the encounter) and elicited countertransference (the reaction induced within the therapist by the service user). Hepple (2011) recognised how confusing transference and countertransference may be as concepts to understand. Perceptions of one another can be formed even prior to the initial engagement (e.g., the service user may have expectations of therapy that are coloured by their friends' experience of therapy; and you as a therapist may have formed a perception of the service user before the first meeting, due to a referral letter or multi-disciplinary team [MDT] discussion). Transference and countertransference feelings can be played out within the therapeutic relationship, and it is here within the middle phase of therapy, when the relationship is more established, that a shared understanding of these issues can emerge through open discussion and use of the map.

Through identifying and discussing patterns within relationships through-out the middle phase of therapy, it is hoped that the therapist is offering a developmentally needed and reparative relationship, replenishing areas which may have been deficient, abusive or overprotective (King, 2005). Having equal-ity within the service user/therapist relationship can encourage adult-to-adult discussion, diminishing feelings of powerlessness and incapability. Such inter-actions can lead to positive reciprocal role identification, which can be mapped through the formation of a 'healthy map' in these mid-sessions.

Considering other models

The beauty of CAT's flexibility and inclusiveness in the middle phase can also feel like an overwhelming and unstructured void for the beginning therapist (hence our attempts to give some structure and guidance in this chapter!) – however we do feel it is important to highlight the ways in which models other than the C and the A can contribute to meaningful change for service users within a cognitive analytic therapy. Many of these have roots in the cognitive behavioural therapies and can be thought of as 'third wave' approaches with slightly different emphases than traditional CBT. We will consider these approaches further below, as alternate offerings to CAT.

As well as crisis management and emotion-regulation strategies, Dialectical Behaviour Therapy (DBT) skills-based interventions are well placed to provide structure for interpersonal effectiveness or 'assertiveness' type interventions, should structure be needed. The assumption underlying this model is that these life- and self-management skills can be useful for absolutely everyone, and that we will all have had varied opportunities to learn these skills during our devel-opmental years. For those of us who did not have an adult around to help us recognise and name our emotions, for example, emotion-recognition skills may be a prerequisite to the work of therapy (and in this way, may need to be con-sidered from the outset).

Karen describes her experiences of recognising her tendency to lose her temper and the work she did on assertiveness:

I found I was still working on that side of me when I came out of therapy really, but she's put [as] the target problem … finding it difficult to deal with pressures from others; I was unable to be assertive and was being too aggressive and had fear of breakdown, obviously that was always sort of connected with those feelings, so in learning how to manage that, and again, I have learnt to be very assertive and I can just say no and no will mean no, and I don't feel like I have to give a reason why I don't want to do something, you know, but I don't have to get like, for instance saying 'well I'll do it' but then being angry with myself and feeling that pres-sure   I always went along – I would just say yes, yes to everything and then once I'd said yes, I'd think no I don't want to do that – then it eats away at you.

Andrew also describes the value of learning the skill of assertion:

Saying no was one of the best words I ever learnt, fantastic, and no and no reason, just no, that's so powerful. The first time I used that I used it by accident – I said no, and I didn't give a reason and they didn't argue with me, and I don't have to do the thing I didn't wanna do – oooh! Oh, this is good, I'm gonna practise this and I'm gonna use that word again and it's quite empowering.

Mindfulness based interventions are a key component of many third wave therapies (most notably, MBCT, DBT, ACT and Compassion Focussed Therapy [CFT]) and can be incredibly helpful in both the recognition and revision phases of CAT (for a more in-depth exploration of the potential relationship between CAT and mindfulness, see Finch, 2013; for a discussion of the differences and tensions between the two approaches, see Marx & Marx, 2012). Additionally, the use of CFT-based interventions (Gilbert, 2010) also lends itself very well to the idea of creating a different relationship with oneself, especially where there are highly self-critical or shame-based procedures at play. The focus upon the felt sense of warmth, connectedness and compassion (often brought alive through imagery work) in CFT can revolutionise treatment where traditional CBT strategies have failed to move heart as well as head.

Lastly, there is growing interest in the use of Eye Movement Desensitisation Reprocessing (EMDR)–based work within CAT approaches, for those who have specific training in this approach. CAT can provide a useful relational frame within which to contain more specific trauma-processing work, with particular reference to complex interpersonal trauma, where this is needed. For example, see Darongkamas et al. (2016) for a consideration of the provision of EMDR within the 'envelope' of CAT.

Healthy mapping in the middle phase

Whilst we would hope to be creating a healthy map (or part maps) from the outset of therapy (as mentioned in Chapter 7), the healthy map can see a flurry of expansion within the middle phase of therapy, as work on revision really gets under way. As Bradley, Cox and Scott (2016) identify, nearly always there is one or more positive relationship within a person's life, whether it be another person, a dog, a cat or even a garden. Thus, in order to give a 'full picture', these relationships too need to be identified throughout the therapy.

Previously, identification of healthy parts of the self was done through adding a 'healthy island' or 'eye-land' to the CAT map and naming such aspects (Nehmad, 1997). The importance of adding the healthy island onto the CAT map was to explicitly show integration between the healthy and less-healthy parts of the self. However, the healthy island was critiqued due to its static nature (e.g., the adding of words, rather than reciprocal roles or procedures) and in relation to the 'unhealthy' parts of the map, it appears visually smaller.

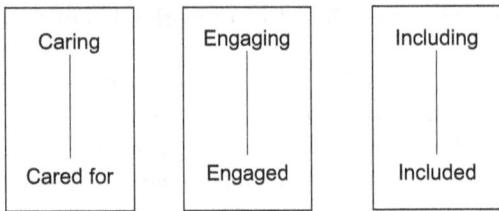

Figure 11.1 Healthy reciprocal roles examples.

Bradley (2012) spoke of the importance of developing a second map, that of a healthy map, to take time to explicitly think of healthy reciprocal roles together, thus modelling the premise that the CAT map is 'not all' of the service user and showing the importance of the healthy self to them.

The middle phase of therapy allows time for this healthy mapping to develop. As the service user begins to recognise and revise problematic patterns, time can be spent thinking about exits and beginning to notice strengths, using these to aid recovery. Bradley et al. (2016) speak of different ways of using a healthy map in the middle phase of therapy. Having a second map to clearly identify healthy roles, which may occur for the service user within relationships outside of therapy (self-to-self or self-to -others), but also within the therapeutic relationship, can be beneficial. Examples of healthy reciprocal roles can be seen in Figure 11.1.

Alternately, Bradley et al. (2016) speak of overlaying the 'strength' reciprocal roles onto the CAT map, using colour coding to highlight different aspects. For example: green to depict strengths, amber to highlight RRs/procedures where there is choice to use an exit/healthy RR or get caught within an unhelpful procedure and red to identify an unmet need or unmanageable feeling. The aim for the service user is not to necessarily avoid the red/amber areas but to find ways of using the green strengths to manage them differently. Many CAT practitioners may find their own style and creativity in identifying healthy RRs and procedures. There is no one way to do this; however, maintaining the premise of including time within the middle phase of therapy to reflect and map healthy aspects is what is most important. Karen shares her healthy map developed within therapy in Figure 11.2.

Link to exits

In considering each of the possible components within the middle stage of CAT, we can see how complex therapy can be, and how important it is to ensure the service user is at the heart of everything we do. Often the most beneficial outcomes are those in which the therapist and service user take time to build their therapeutic relationship, and the service user feels invested within the therapy, involved within the development of the CAT map and dialogical understandings and engaged within working through difficult situations outside of the therapy setting. We have formed an appreciation that it is the interaction between the

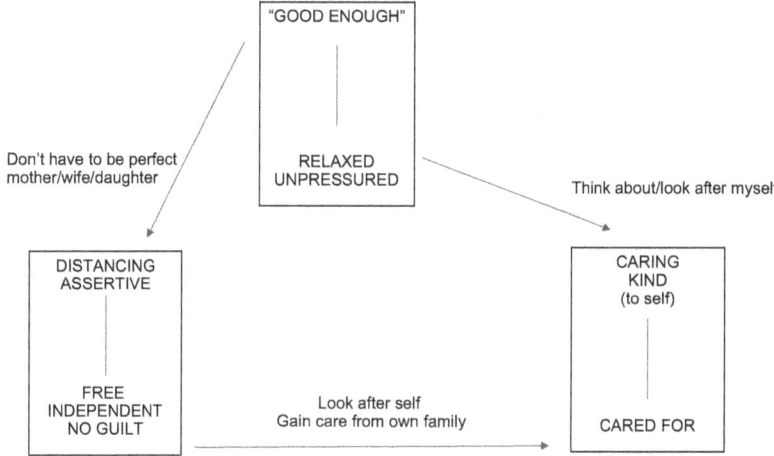

EXIT: I can deal with pressure from others by being assertive, keeping some distance and not feeling guilty about it.

Figure 11.2 Karen's healthy map.

therapist and service user in recognising problematic patterns together that can lead to forming an understanding of how to step out of them, leading to the revision phase of CAT. These adaptations that the service user can make to the thought, behaviour or relational interaction are called exits. Exits can be identified at any stage throughout the therapeutic contract and can be recorded together within sessions. We will explore the process of developing exits together in the next chapter. Here, Karen and Andrew share their experiences of therapy and how they began to take steps forward in their own wellbeing.

Karen says:

> *...there were some weeks I would want to run into therapy because something that had happened in the week and I really wanted to share it and I really wanted to offload it so there were some days I was running there and wanted to talk it through with them and make some sense of it.*

Andrew says:

> *I think all the other therapies that helped as well because you kind of say that the more you put in, the more you get out. Therapy was always hard work; you know it was always whatever day I went and had therapy that was the day written off, possibly the day after written off, so it was anything that's going to be worth it is going to be hard work so I think that's what got me going back and also you know feeling guilty of I've been given this opportunity and I've got to see it through.*

Conclusion

The middle phase of therapy is individualised for every service user and is person-centred, based upon the developing CAT map and service user need. Often, the CAT practitioner has their own preferred ways of working (e.g., they may lean more towards the C rather than the A in CAT or vice versa), including drawing upon different approaches. The integrative nature of CAT allows the therapist to consider ways to assist the service user in stepping out of their problematic procedures, for example, through the use of compassion focussed therapy or mindfulness, as discussed. Finally, the ultimate aim of the middle phase of therapy is to begin to develop exits to problematic patterns and to begin to develop a healthy map, allowing the service user space to recognise their strengths and protective factors, alongside how to maintain these.

References

Bennett, D. (1995). The use of transference in CAT: Refinement of a proposed model. *Reformulation*, Spring.

Bradley, J. (2012). A hopeful sequential diagrammatic. *Reformulation*, Summer, 13–15.

Bradley, J., Cox, P., & Scott, J. (2016). A hopeful sequential diagrammatic reformulation - Four years on. *Reformulation*, Summer, 33–38.

Darongkamas, J., Kiely, B., & Walker, M. J. (2016). A CAT envelope to deliver EMDR: Cognitive Analytic Therapy around eye movement desensitization and reprocessing. *Journal of Psychotherapy Integration*, 26(4), 462–477. https://psycnet.apa.org/doi/10.1037/int0000034

Finch, J. (2013). CAT in dialogue with mindfulness: Thoughts on a theoretical and clinical integration. *Reformulation*, 41, 45–48.

Gilbert, P. (2010). *Compassion Focused Therapy: Distinctive Features*. Taylor & Francis.

Hepple, J. (2011). The Chicken and The Egg. *Reformulation*, Winter, 19.

King, R. (2005). CAT, the therapeutic relationship and working with people with learning disability. *Reformulation*, Spring, 10–14.

Koons, C. R. (2016). *How to handle the doorknob comment*. https://www.newharbinger.com/blog/quick-tips-therapists/how-to-handle-the-doorknob-comment/

Marx, R. & Marx, S. (2012). The eye and the 'I': The construction and use of the observer in Cognitive–Analytic Psychotherapy and mindfulness-based therapy. *British Journal of Psychotherapy*, 28(4), 496–515. https://doi.org/10.1111/j.1752-0118.2012.01308.x

Nehmad, A. (1997). Beyond state shifts-metashifts. *Reformulation, ACAT News*, Summer.

Ryle, A. & Kerr, I. (2020). *Introducing Cognitive Analytic Therapy. Principles and Practice of a Relational Approach to Mental Health*. Wiley.

12 Exits and doing something different

Introduction

Within this chapter we focus on the revision stage of CAT, the phase in which we begin to identify and discuss change. We consider the term 'exit' within the framework of CAT, alongside how to recognise and record exits which are identified. In addition, we discuss the differing types of exits that can be facilitated and observed and offer a model of exits for us as developing clinicians to hold in mind. Finally, we focus on consolidation and maintenance of change over time.

Conceptualising and recognising exits

First and foremost, a word on language. The term *exit* in CAT refers to anything that allows the service user to move away from or step out of a problematic pattern. This might be an 'internal' shift in thoughts, feelings and understandings or a more externally observable, behavioural change. Whilst we do use the term 'exit' to refer to these shifts and changes with our service users, it is worth noting that this language may have different connotations or meanings for different people. For some, the term 'exit' may have associations with more damaging forms of escape, such as suicide and serious self-harm. As always, then, it is prudent to check out with your service user how they feel about this term, what it might mean or be associated with for them, and whether they would prefer a different term to refer to these positive steps away from what has been keeping them stuck.

As we've outlined above, an exit can be anything that entails doing, perceiving or experiencing something differently from the problematic patterns and roles that have been identified through the process of CAT reformulation and mapping. They are necessarily varied in nature and often idiosyncratic to the individual service user (Toye, 2009). Bear in mind that exits can be planned behavioural changes/experiments, agreed in advance during therapy sessions, or implicit and somewhat unconscious shifts that the service user may not even be initially aware of. Toye (2009) describes the latter as spontaneous discoveries, which may happen at any stage of therapy. Exits can also be experienced in

DOI: 10.4324/9781003308256-12

the therapy room between therapist and service user. Here the therapist may resist a pull to join the dance within a problematic procedure, and as a result, a different position may be found.

Exits may constitute changes in how the service user relates to themselves, or in how they relate to others; and, perhaps most importantly, they can be seemingly the smallest steps and still be of huge significance to the person you're working with. We mention this mostly to remind ourselves of the adage that 'comparison is the thief of joy', that the pressure of expectation can leave both us and our service users failing to recognise and celebrate the value of those first few tentative steps in what will inevitably be a life-long journey.

Karen describes here how her therapist highlighted her core difficulties in the centre of the map, explaining both the problem patterns that these resulted in and the exits that emerged from them:

Karen says:

> *In the middle of everything she put that I wasn't cared for and that my needs were not being met and that nobody was looking after me. Manifesting into me trying to be the perfect wife, the perfect mother, the perfect daughter. Again, striving and feeling pressured. But then the exit from that was learning that I'm good enough and that everything I do is good enough. That's when she put: 'things don't have to be perfect, and I don't have to be perfect'. Again, the criticising/ neglecting was how I felt with myself as well. So, it had come from feeling neglected and uncared for and then I was starting to criticise and neglect myself, but the exit from that was the relaxing 'me' time and learning to focus more on myself and staying calm and talking to people calmly and being assertive rather than being the angry person that I was 'cos I used to very, very easily lose my temper.*

Developing and recognising exits

Similar to the middle phase of therapy, exits have not been covered to a great extent in the literature. This may be because exits are individual to the service user and based upon their own problematic patterns and experiences of how to step out of them. As a result, it is difficult therefore to guide the developing therapist in the 'how-to' of exits within therapy. Whilst exits can come naturally from recognition, we can begin to conceptualise them through considering their differing presentations. We present here our multidimensional model of exits to aim to introduce the distinctive features that can be noted when identifying ways out of problematic patterns (see Figure 12.1).

The two dimensions of the model comprise that of 'implicit to explicit' and 'internal to external'. The former dimension relates to how far exits are planned, with 'implicit' being more suggestive of natural change occurring ad hoc and, in the moment, whereas 'explicit' denotes intentionally tested-out exits. The latter, 'internal to external', refers to the locus of change, where

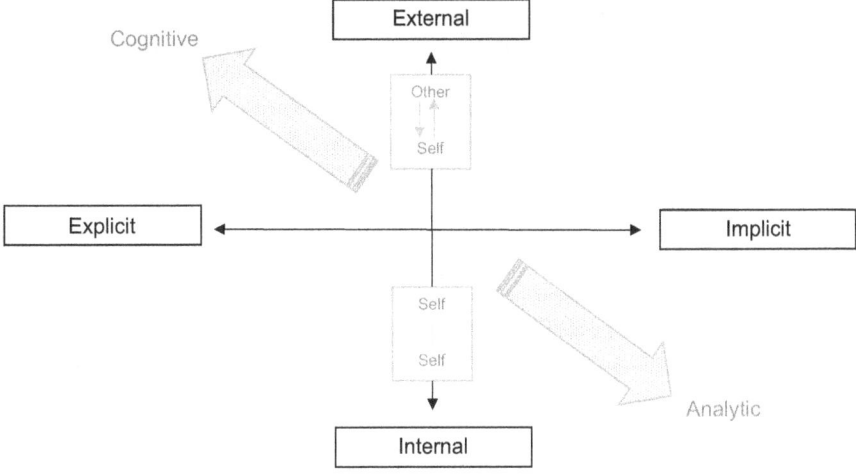

Figure 12.1 Model of exits.

'internal' suggests an emotional shift within the service user (self-to-self), whilst 'external' symbolises behavioural change which is outwardly observable both to the service user and to others (others-to-self and self-to-others).

The following highlights the exits that can be observed at each of the four ends of the dimensions in more detail.

Explicit and external exits

When the explicit and external dimensions come together, the service user and therapist will be working towards active change. They will agree together on testing out an explicit hypothesis (such as suggesting a behavioural change to a specific trap or dilemma). Behavioural experiments can often be discussed within the session, and the service user can then actively work on the change outside of the sessions. Graded exposure can be an example of this, where the service user can work on differing levels of change over the course of the middle phase of therapy. In doing so, the service user can observe change which they have made, which is also noticeable to others. Alongside the behavioural change, a cognitive shift may also come with time.

Explicit and internal exits

Explicit, internal changes made within the therapy are also intentional, deliberate attempts at doing something different. The difference in this case, however, is that the service user experiences an emotional change within the self, leading to a self-to-self exit. Here, such planned opportunities to make change can include interventions such as mindfulness, self-imagery and aiding self-compassion.

The aim with these exits is to shift the service user's relationship with negative thinking and to create a more compassionate relationship with the self.

Implicit and external exits

In this end of the continuum, the service user may experience the opportunity to make change outside of the therapy and takes it. Once again, the exit is external, and thus observable to the self and others; however, the change is implicit, occurring ad hoc and naturally, in the moment as the opportunity arises. Often, these exits are understood and reflected on through discussion with therapist in retrospect. Examples of such exits can be through altering an interaction with another person by adapting behaviour to elicit an alternate response.

Implicit and internal exits

Exits which usually take time to occur within the therapy are the implicit and internal shifts. This is due to the change being internalised and a greater self-to-self emotional shift occurring. These exits are often identified within a session, when a service user makes a reflection on their own self-to-self relationship, such as 'I know I am not all to blame'. These times in therapy often feel like a 'win', as the emotional shift for the service user is noted and the deepness of change is reflected upon. This end of the two dimensions often draws upon the analytic theory, with relational interactions being paramount, as the service user works towards healthier reciprocal roles, such as caring-to-cared-for.

Recording exits

As exits are identified within sessions, it is important to make sure that they are captured in some way, enabling the service user to notice their progression and change over time. In addition, through the recording of exits, a tool is created which the service user is then able to keep and use once therapy comes to an end, as a reminder of ways in which they did things differently and stepped out of their problematic patterns.

Generally, there is no strict rule or guidance as to how the therapist supports the service user in recording these exits, and this can be done in a number of ways throughout sessions, depending on therapist preference or service user's choice. Some examples of such recording, however, can be to have a key and list; writing the exit on the map; building the healthy map or colour-coding the map. We will take a moment to expand on each of these in more detail:

1. *The key and list.* Here the therapist will guide the service user to think about where on their map they have exited and identify this with a number (working in numerical order as exits are recognised). The number is written

directly on the map where the exit has occurred, following which a narrative of how the service user has made the change is written on a separate sheet, alongside its corresponding number. It is important to work collaboratively with the service user using their words to explain the exit, as this captures the essence of the exit and can aid further recognition in the future when used outside of the therapy.

2. *On the map*. Some therapists find it most useful to depict the exit on the map (for example see Karen's map, Figure 9.10, in Chapter 9). Here an arrow is written to highlight where the exit is occurring, and key words are used to highlight what the exit comprises of.

3. *Building the healthy map*. As we have mentioned in previous chapters, the healthy map is important within the therapy to identify alternate ways of being and more positive patterns and reciprocal roles (see Karen's healthy map, Figure 11.2 in Chapter 11, for an example of this). It is also a useful way of recording exits, as through discussion of how the service user has done something different, you can identify together healthy ways of relating.

4. *Colour coding*. Bradley et al. (2016) speak of the use of colour-coding on maps, with red being used to depict unmet need/unmanageable feelings; amber highlighting procedures where there is a choice to move and identify an exit or become caught within the RRP; and green where successful exits are sought.

What if change doesn't come?

The experience of many CAT therapists and service user's is that once good enough, in-the-moment recognition occurs, change follows naturally. However, this is certainly not always the case, and we wouldn't want to perpetuate an idea of 'perfect, textbook-style' therapy – because of course, there is no such thing! Sometimes recognition is present but change remains stubbornly elusive. There can be many reasons for this, and again, it would be seriously remiss of us to encourage you to assume that they are all situated within the service user, or indeed the therapeutic relationship, as external factors often form the most potent barriers to change. We shall, however, give some consideration to what we do know about the process of change in CAT – how this is experienced and understood, and what might facilitate or impede this, with the aim of providing some food for thought for the times when things do become stuck.

Let's consider what we know about the service user's experience of change within CAT. Rayner et al. (2011) were among the first authors to look explicitly at how people who've received CAT relate their experience of change to the main therapeutic tools of the approach. They completed 15 semi-structured interviews with nine service users who had received CAT and used a grounded theory approach to analyse the resultant data. The core framework that all other categories seemed to relate to within this study was the idea of 'doing with' – the working relationship between service user and therapist – and more specifically, the idea that therapy is hard work; you can't just 'sit back and let it happen' as one participant put it; you have to work *alongside* your therapist. Subsumed within this framework were the sub-categories of 'being with the therapist', 'understanding and feeling', 'keeping it real' and 'CAT tools'. The category of 'being with the therapist' encapsulated all those qualities that you'd hope a good therapeutic relationship would foster (trust, feeling valued, safe and secure) – in particular, there seemed to be an important sense of *feeling free to express painful emotions and having confidence that the therapist could help to contain this.* The category of 'understanding and feeling' referred to the idea of needing to *go through the discomfort associated with painful emotions* (a 'necessary evil') *in order to gain understanding* and therefore step back and access choices about doing things differently. Interestingly, all participants expressed the belief that therapy is 'not a cure' and acknowledged that their (long-standing) patterns were still there and could be re-triggered by external events in the future – change is a 'continuous' process that therapy can only ever open the door to. The category of 'keeping it real' related to the importance of *'doing...and not just talking'* – using practical tools and working on everyday examples helped to facilitate this. The fourth category, 'CAT tools', linked in with each of the previous three – of particular note was the observation that those who had the *strongest emotional reactions to the tools and took an active role in co-constructing them appeared to gain the most benefit from them.* These authors conclude that the role of feelings in CAT is key – affective arousal is needed as well as insight to bring about change.

Interestingly, this has echoes with both Karen's and Andrew's description of CAT – their sessions felt like an emotional roller-coaster at times, which they often felt the pull to withdraw from. However, with their continued engagement and ability to stay with the emotional experience of therapy, they were able to reap its rewards. Perhaps most relevant to our current purposes, the authors reflect on the gradual and sometimes erratic process of change – whilst some participants recalled feeling stuck at points in their therapy, in hindsight all service users reflected that change had been occurring at these times – this relates to the previous point we made about the importance of recognising small changes.

Next, we consider how therapists collaborate with service users in developing exits. Sandhu et al. (2017) used qualitative content analysis on audio recordings of therapy sessions from eight participants who were receiving CAT for depression. The main categories of 'exit work' that they uncovered were (1) development of an observing self, (2) change in procedures and roles and (3) support and maintenance of change. The first category described the processes by which the service user increased their capacity for self-reflection – the main ways that this seemed to happen were through *feedback from the therapist* ('therapist facilitated recognition') and through *observations that the service users were able to make themselves.* These related both to 'out of session' and 'in session' material – although it was noted that only the therapists initiated reflections on 'in session' enactments within the therapeutic relationship. The category of 'change in procedures and roles' involved service users trying out new or re-engaging with previous, positive roles and procedures, both self-to-self and self-to-other. In particular, these were summarised as *self-care, being assertive, self-compassion* (for example by resisting patterns of being self-critical) and *using motivating self-talk*. The final category, 'support and maintenance of change' involved the therapists scaffolding change. This involved *planning exits to be tried within the service user's ZPD, identifying proposed exits using the SDR, attending to the process and feelings associated with change, recognition of and encouragement in relation to changes made* and *prompting thinking about the maintenance of exits via the goodbye letter*. This study aimed to add to our understanding of how CAT therapists enable change in collaboration with service users. In fact, many of the categories are reflected in our dialogue with Karen and Andrew – in particular the process of therapists initially scaffolding recognition with service users, the use of self-care, self-compassion and assertiveness as exits (explicit and internal exits) and the prompts for ongoing work in the goodbye letter. The overall framework of understanding change as interconnected phases of "reflection, action and consolidation" (Sandhu et al., 2017, p. 1270) may be especially helpful to beginning CAT therapists both as a guide for when things become stuck and as a prompt to consider the foundations for consolidation of exits.

The consolidation of exits

Change can take time. The initial developments of exits within the therapy room are important to document and reflect upon together, using the map, so that the service user is clear on how they have stepped out of the problematic pattern. Through having such conversations, the therapist is working towards deepening reflection and recognition in the hope that in the future the service user will be able to notice and exit from problematic patterns on their own, outside of therapy. As the service user works towards the end of therapy, they may discuss with the therapist ways in which to continue to make change. On occasion, the therapist may suggest internalising their voice, for example, *'when this happens, think about what we have spoken about in therapy and what my response may have been'*. At times, due to the strength of the therapeutic relationship, this might come naturally for the service user, and they may find they often think back to what was said in sessions. Karen gives a useful example of this from her own experience:

Karen says:

> *I've also stepped back and I don't criticise myself the way I used to; I was always my biggest enemy really, criticising myself and then I think yeah but, you don't deserve the criticism and why are you being like that? Again it's learned, it's learned from trying to be that perfect child and it's detaching, but yeah, I think her [therapist] voice, it's her voice that comes into my head – like what would she say in this scenario? "What is it you're trying to achieve"? And you don't wanna do that so what're you doing it for then?*

Using reciprocal roles, we can consider such internalisation from a CAT perspective (thus developing implicit, internal exits). As therapy comes to an end, we may reflect with the service user about how they are becoming 'their own therapist', through questioning their own behaviour, having space to think about it and considering change. As therapists ourselves, we have often suggested to our own service users about having some dedicated time to do this in the first instance, following the contract of therapy coming to an end. This may be through maintaining the same day and time each week that the CAT sessions were held, for the service user to have space to review the week and reflect upon any progress made.

Karen speaks to this in her own reflections:

> *I can always remember even my consultant, 'cos I used to always depend on my son for those talks to bring me back if you like to who I am expressing all my, like, worries to him. And I remember my consultant saying you will learn to have those conversations with yourself. When he's gone off and got married and that. And he said, well you will learn that. How do you learn that but you do? Yeah. And I find myself even now when I walk the dog having [those] conversations in your head where's those thoughts coming from? What's that about? Like rationalising.*

Having space with Karen and Andrew to discuss their experiences of CAT some 10–12 years ago, alongside noting that our own therapy was similarly this long ago, has been useful in thinking about the longevity of CAT. For the four of us, we still continue to reflect upon and use our CAT maps today and have continued to develop exits to our problematic patterns over the last decade. We all may continue to fall into our traps at times, but having a map within our mind of our own procedures allows us to consider and use exits. Karen describes here her recognition of the need to keep working on the ways in which her more angry feelings were expressed beyond the end of her CAT sessions:

Karen says:

> *I knew at the time when my therapy come to an end that was something I was gonna have to still continue to work on, and I do, and I don't recognise that person now, that person isn't there who'd be like running about the house like an idiot being angry 'cos it's exhausting as well, not to say you are perfect or you don't lose your temper, of course you do, but you realise by talking and sharing how you feel it's so more effective isn't it than losing it.*

As we move through therapy and the service user begins to identify exits to the problematic patterns, it is important to continue to reflect on how they are making progress themselves, outside of the therapy. This is necessary as we will see next within the 'Saying Goodbye' chapter, as not only does the service user need to experience what it's like to come to an end, but they also need to encounter time outside of therapy, to be able to 'go it alone' and recognise their own skills and strengths in applying exits within their day to day life.

Conclusion

The process of change in CAT is one which often comes with time, space to reflect, development of the observing eye and the service user's readiness to do something different. Exits can be developed both through explicit and implicit processes, within and outside of the therapy room. Having space within the therapy to discuss the ways in which the service user has made change and to record these in written format allows for further consolidation of change. When change is slower or there is a feeling of 'stuckness' within the room, revisiting the map to discuss what such feelings may be about is useful. On occasion, change can be minimal; however through engaging within the process of CAT, the service user leaves with differing knowledge about themselves and others, to what they had when coming into therapy. At other times, change can be significant, and the service user wholeheartedly feels a difference within themselves and to their wellbeing.

References

Bradley, J., Cox, P., & Scott, P. (2016). A hopeful sequential diagrammatic reformulation – Four years on. *Reformulation*, Summer, 30–39.

Rayner, K., Thompson, A. R., & Walsh, S. (2011). Clients' experience of the process of change in cognitive analytic therapy. *Psychology and Psychotherapy: Theory, Research and Practice*, 84, 299–313. https://doi.org/10.1348/147608310x531164

Sandhu, S. K., Kellett, S., & Hardy, G. (2017). The development of a change model of "exits" during cognitive analytic therapy for the treatment of depression. *Clinical Psychology and Psychotherapy*, 24(6), 1263–1272. https://doi.org/10.1002/cpp.2090

Toye, J. (2009). Aims and exits from self-defeating procedures. *Reformulation*, Summer, 26–29.

13 Saying goodbye

Introduction

Cognitive Analytic Therapy (CAT) fundamentally considers the ending from the start of the therapy, and thus, the therapist needs to be mindful throughout of any difficulties which may arise as the sessions come to a close. This chapter will explore the 'how- to' of preparing for an ending, writing a goodbye letter and collaborating with the service user in the final session to say goodbye. Considerations will then be made as to what happens following the ending, leading us into contemplating the 'journey beyond the therapy room'.

When does the ending begin?

As touched upon already in previous chapters, the ending is always at the forefront of the therapist's mind, given that CAT is a time-limited, structured and contracted approach. Whilst we consider the 'saying goodbye' part of the process as something which occurs in the latter half of the contract, it is important to name the ending from the beginning, within the early stages of contracting with the service user. The choice of the number of sessions (e.g., 8, 12, 16 or 24) will have been based on what length of time the service user is anticipated to require within therapy, in order to facilitate a 'good enough' ending. Mann (1973) spoke of the importance of setting an ending at the beginning of therapy, regardless of what the service user's previous experience of loss is.

Jellema (1999) spoke frequently about the importance of the use of attachment within CAT, where the therapist models a secure relationship from which the service user can then explore their exits and come back to the therapy to discuss them. The therapist elicits such scaffolding to provide a safe base whilst allowing for complex thinking about loss and the emotional impact the service user may experience as a result. Therefore, discussions can be held as they arise, throughout the therapeutic process, and tentative connections can be made to the ending of therapy and what this may feel like for the service user. For some service users, loss may be a significant part of the CAT map, and thus it will be important throughout the therapy to work on exits and identify how these exits can be used as the final session approaches.

DOI: 10.4324/9781003308256-13

As mentioned in Chapter 11, the 'counting down' of therapy sessions is also a way of recognising time within the therapy with the service user and indicating when the ending will occur. The discussion surrounding the 'middle point' of therapy can also trigger feelings surrounding how quickly time has passed and how near the ending is as it approaches. It allows for open exploration of ways in which endings can be difficult, any fears the service user may have with regards to the ending (e.g., not having achieved sufficient; feeling abandoned, to name two) and what the focus may be for the remaining sessions. Towards the latter end of the therapy, the therapist may enable further discussion about the feelings in relation to the ending as it approaches, and how together the therapist and service user can work towards a 'healthier', 'safer', 'good enough' ending, which may be different from what the service user has experienced in the past. Andrew shares what it was like for him facing the ending of the sessions with his therapist.

Andrew says:

> *I was joking to my wife about coming towards the end of therapy sessions and it was like junior school where you take your toys in and play for the last day it's gonna be one of them. And I came out and it was like 'what the hell happened to you?' It was like 'I didn't bring my toys in, it wasn't like that'. That was really deep and that was really, really hard.*
>
> *And I don't think strict is the right word, but she was at that side which was attachment, which I needed, erm, I kind of had abandonment issues so every time I finished therapy I was like I'm not gonna see them and I'm gonna be on my own again and that didn't feel that because we knew from the start you know and she'd mention 'right we're at week 7' or whatever and the goodbye letter.*

How do I prepare for the ending?

Preparation for the ending takes place inside and outside of the therapy room, both for the service user and the therapist. Some therapists prefer to share their goodbye letter in the final session, whereas others may choose to do this in the penultimate session (with space in the last session for any final thoughts). Penultimate session letters can often be planned, if there is a strong hypothesis that the service user is unlikely to attend the final session, due to fearing the ending, or saying goodbye.

When it is planned for the goodbye letters to be shared within the final session, usually the penultimate session is when letters are discussed and a structure for the final session is made. In the penultimate session, the therapist can share with the service user the importance of marking the ending and consider the reciprocal nature of the giving of a goodbye letter. Hamill et al. (2008) hypothesised that goodbye letters help service users cope better with termination and provide a record of the therapeutic process that they can keep through the follow-up and beyond. It can be a way of reflecting on the ending, what has been achieved, and the relationship, whilst also acknowledging loss and disappointment. Hamill et al. (2008) noted that service users often identified feeling able to say things within their own goodbye letters that they wouldn't have been able to previously.

It is important for the therapist to discuss with the service user the invitation for them to write a goodbye letter to the therapist, with an aim to share it within the final session. The service user can be provided with a very simple, written brief, to guide the writing of the goodbye letter. This can comprise a sentence or two such as:

> *Within the final session, I would like you to come with a letter to share, explaining your experience of therapy, what you have learnt and where it leaves you now. I will do the same.*

It is important for the service user to be made aware that the goodbye letter is not a prerequisite for attending. If they struggle with writing the letter in any way, it is preferable that they feel comfortable in returning to the final session without one, so the ending can continue to be processed together. In addition, as not all service users enjoy writing, it can often be helpful to offer alternate ways to express their goodbye (e.g., through a picture or poem).

How might I feel as a therapist saying goodbye to the service user?

Alongside being aware of the impact of the ending on the service user, it is also important to consider your own emotions, as these will differ for each service user you see. As you write your goodbye letter, it is important to take a step back and think about how you are feeling in relation to the ending: do you feel a sense of sadness, or anxiety at how the service user will cope, or do you feel cut off from any feelings? As you think about these emotions, it is then worth thinking about whether these may belong to you or to the service user. Knowing yourself in CAT is important, as you can then reflect on what you bring to the therapy. For example, if you struggle with endings and separations, you may find that your anxiety increases as the final session approaches, or that you feel a pull to want to offer more. Alternately, if you are feeling a different emotion to what you normally would as an ending approaches, it is worth considering whether this is a projection from the service user (e.g., you feel a sense of abandonment and despair that the ending is coming and are concerned for the service user's wellbeing outside of the therapy. This could belong to the service user, as they worry about how to navigate life outside of the weekly, routine sessions).

Martin and Schurtman (1985) spoke broadly about the anxiety and apprehension that a therapist may feel as they come to the ending of therapy. They identified five sources of termination anxiety, which they highlighted as follows:

1. *Termination dynamics which are independent of the service user reaction.* This is the time in which the feelings may come from your own personal history of endings. Martin and Schurtman (1985) suggest that if a therapist has incomplete separation from his or her own parent in childhood, they may be more vulnerable to separation anxiety from the service user, and thus struggle with the ending.
2. *Anxiety over the loss of the professional role during termination.* Here it is proposed that there comes a point at the end of therapy, where the professional relationship comes to an end (e.g., the service user is no longer the service user and the therapist is no longer the therapist). Therefore, new identities within the relationship need to be formed.
3. *Therapist's reaction to the service user's termination anxiety.* This is where the therapist may experience projection of the service user's response to the ending, which can include a host of feelings such as anger, abandonment, sadness, denial, joy, rejection and guilt.
4. *Uneasiness of the implied importance of termination.* The therapist may feel an 'overconcern' in ensuring that the therapy ends successfully. The ending can be a time where further growth for the service user occurs; therefore, the therapist can feel an increase in anxiety to ensure it goes well.
5. *Literal loss of a meaningful relationship.* If a trusting, engaging and collaborative relationship has been formed throughout the therapy, the therapist may feel a huge sense of loss, in terms of working with a service user where the work has been rewarding.

Whilst the Martin and Schurtman (1985) paper is now nearly 40 years old, the considerations that are made in terms of termination anxiety for the therapist are still pertinent. There may be certain areas of termination that the therapist finds themselves more naturally thinking about than others (e.g., the service user's feelings and the loss of the relationship). Less so, the therapist may find themselves thinking about their own loss of professional role (from a personal reflective perspective, as the professional relationship is then complete), particularly due to the fast pace of endings and new beginnings within the professional setting.

How do I write a goodbye letter?

As with reformulation letter writing, time is needed in advance of the final session for the therapist to reflect upon the content of sessions and to write the goodbye letter. The goodbye letter can take time to write, and the therapist will require a boundaried, quiet space and sufficient time to do this. In short, Ryle (1997) summarised the content of the goodbye letter as being 'what has been achieved and what remains to be done'. The suggested content of the goodbye letter has been well documented within the literature, with Ryle and Kerr (2002) first providing structure. They suggested that the letter should include:

- an accurate, plain and unvarnished summary of the therapy;
- a summary of original problems and procedures, with consideration of how these have been resolved;
- identification of what future work is required;
- consideration of how the person has been open to accept help and how that which has been valued can be retained;
- how the ending feels, including potential disappointment, sadness and anger;
- positive achievements and a reminder of developed conceptual tools;
- attending to uncertainties or unresolved feelings.

Turpin et al. (2011) completed a study to consider what Inter-Regional Residential ACAT Psychotherapy Training (IRRAPT) trainees find are important ingredients of a goodbye letter. Through auditing 20 returned questionnaires (with a 90% response rate), they developed the following mnemonic, to help therapists remember the key contents of the letter.

F – feelings and endings
A – achievements
R – relationship
E – expression of hope
W – warm and engaging
E – exits
L – language used
L – life/learning after therapy

Having written a number of goodbye letters between us throughout our careers, we too can identify with this mnemonic and the importance of these key ingredients. It is vital to remember that the goodbye letter is not a repeat of the reformulation letter. It is not there to repeat the problematic patterns fully, and indeed for some service users (those for who feeling criticised has been a particularly painful place, for example), it may be more validating to get to a sense of what has been achieved as soon as possible. The letter does, however, aim to highlight the therapeutic relationship, any threats to the alliance and how ruptures were managed, as well as exits identified within sessions. The letter should talk about the review, and what the journey outside of the therapy may be like for the service user. Closing the letter with a final statement about your own feelings? About the ending can be useful, for example: Will you miss them? Can you thank them for their genuineness/openness?

Once you have completed the letter, it is important to take it to supervision to share. This will give you practice of reading through the letter prior to sharing it within the session, but also will allow you to have a discussion with your supervisor about its contents and any amendments that are required. Once changes have been made, you can then print two copies, ready for sharing within the final session, considering creative means of sharing the goodbye letter with the service user, if needed. Here, Karen has shared the goodbye letter she received from her therapist at the end of therapy. Karen's therapist has also provided consent for this to be shared. Names have been removed from the letter to maintain confidentiality. Following the letter, Karen goes on to share her reflections on saying goodbye and receiving the letter within the final session.

Karen's Goodbye Letter from Therapist

This is a therapeutic letter not to be taken out of the context of CAT

Dear Karen,
We have reached the end of your 16 sessions of therapy. This letter aims to summarise the things we have talked about and what we have learned, as well as identifying the exits you have made. There are also things you can continue to work on and think about until we meet for our follow-up appointment. It has been quite a ride for you! There have been ups and downs, and some difficult realisations, but you have worked really hard and stuck with it, so well done!

You came to therapy with a need to resolve issues from the past. You felt you were perhaps taking things out on mum, feeling increasingly snappy and irritated with her and her demands. You wanted to have a better relationship with her (but minus the demands) particularly as she is quite elderly now.

There was also a need to be more relaxed in life generally. You feared stress as you related this to having a breakdown and this connected to memories of hospital admissions. Your target problem was about the difficulty in dealing with pressure from others.

Over the course of therapy, you have successfully detached from mum, not an easy task after a lifetime of being 'strangulated' and stifled by her. There is a new reciprocal role of distancing/assertive – free/independent/guiltless. Mum did not react well at first, becoming in your words, more demanding and manipulating. Initially you felt very guilty about being assertive, saying no and doing things on your terms, but this guilt has subsided over time. You have come to realise that it is perfectly acceptable to think about yourself. Obviously, you would not see harm come to your mother, but you know what she is and isn't capable of doing.

Unfortunately, as you did less for her, mum seemed to shut you out which has been very hurtful. You still wanted to have contact, share phone calls and have some closeness, just not have to meet every demand, but it seems as though mum is only interested if you are 'useful' to her.

Another complicating factor was the reconnection with your sister. You wrote her a letter after having had no contact for four years. You hoped for a supportive relationship, someone to 'share the burden' of mother. It was a little bumpy at first. The more your sister became involved, the less contact you had with mum, as your sister took on your old role and met mum's demands. This was where the realisation came that you would not have the close mother/daughter relationship you would like and that perhaps you were not as special to her as she had made you believe.

I think you have been really strong to stand your ground. Feeling neglected could have made you feel quite clingy, and you might have been drawn back into the old pattern of meeting demands, to feel wanted. But you are keeping your distance.

Things with your sister also seem to have settled. You are both aware that mum can 'play you off' and you both take what she says about the other with a pinch of salt. Your sister has realised what you have had to deal with over the years. She has confirmed the neglect from your childhood, and there is a shared history and understanding which allows you to take care of one another. There is another new reciprocal role of caring/kind to cared for. This is essentially what you wanted from mum, but in understanding that this is unlikely to happen, you have become more open to your sister.

In other areas of your life, you are also trying to think about letting go of pressures. We realised that you had a tendency to strive and that things had to be perfect. You would do lots and lots of chores on your days off but feel resentful that there was never any time for yourself, but you feared criticism and felt guilty if you didn't do it.

It sounds as though you have embraced the idea of good enough! (good enough to relaxed/unpressured). You are able to challenge thoughts around not being perfect and are finding time to relax and think about yourself. You are also not taking it personally if your husband wants to do housework. It is not a criticism of you, but something he likes to do.

In taking the pressure off and relaxing a little, you are essentially being kind and caring to yourself. You can then extend this care to your own family, because you are not feeling stressed and snappy.

To summarise, I think the main thing to work on is the relationship with your mother. We have talked in length about how you can maintain contact with her perhaps by only phoning a few times per week. Keeping some distance and maintaining your independence is important. Accepting mum for who she is (rather than what you want her to be) is also important.

We know now that your mum is unlikely to provide you with the care and attention you would like, and which has been missing all your life. It is up to you now to decide whether this is acceptable and how much work you want to put into the relationship, bearing in mind you will likely get little back.

It is all the more important to continue to think about yourself. Take time to relax and be kind and caring to yourself. If anyone else is making demands, remember to be assertive and say 'no' when you really don't want to do something.

Perhaps anger is something to work on too. You are fiery and emotional by nature, and when emotions are running high, it feels difficult to restrain your reactions. However, you have realised that you are less volatile now and arguments that have cropped up with your husband have been much better managed. Continue to work on this. Practice taking a deep breath so you can think before you speak. Walk away from a situation if you must and then approach it again when you are calmer.

I wish you all the best, Karen. It has been lovely to work with you. You have invested a lot of time and energy in the therapy and come a long way. I hope you continue to reap the rewards of this.

I would suggest we meet in eight weeks' time. Have a lovely Christmas. Best Wishes,
[therapist]

Karen says:

Do you know what did strike me, it's that letter at the end, the ending was just so perfect. Summarising to me and what I've been through she just hit it perfect. And then when you read it back it's emotional and when you read that final letter back and you think yeah that's what I presented with and that's me. It's very hard hitting that letter at the end. It felt funny when I looked at those, no it's not me, it's like 10–11 years ago you know and you know what I thought was amazing I had to get in touch with her about something and in the message I was telling her what I did at uni and I mean this is after 13 years and she said, 'Karen that's absolutely perfect for you, ah not perfect, I mean good enough'! Wow for you to like remember that after 13 years and it's the key thing I've took away from it, that's the best bit.

Sharing the goodbye letter

Within the session you have mutually agreed to share the goodbye letter, you will start the session by acknowledging the ending has arrived, and checking in with the service user about how they are feeling about this. It is helpful to return to the plan to share goodbye letters with one another, and to see if the service user has been able to write one of their own. You may consider with the service user what their preferences are as to who reads the letter first. This can alleviate any anxieties for the service user, as sometimes they report wanting to get it 'over and done with' and at other times they prefer wanting to hear the therapist's letter first (due to anticipatory anxiety about its contents). Whatever their decision, this is the order you will go with, with regards to sharing the letter within the session. Hamill et al. (2008) recognised that most service users experienced anxiety in sharing their own letters as they were not sure what was expected or whether it would be good enough.

For the purpose of the following example, we will consider the service user giving their letter first. It is important to ensure the service user feels safe and happy enough to read their letter within the session. Then, provide the service user with guidance, handing over to them to read the letter through to you. Within the moment, listen carefully to the contents of the letter. It is often helpful to explore with the service user how they had found writing the letter, what they had wanted to include/not include and how they are feeling now in having shared the letter with you. Following on from this, you can then suggest the sharing of your letter. With having two letters printed off, you will be able to provide one copy to the service user to follow along with you whilst you read from your copy. If you are working online with a service user, ask them whether or not they would like the letter sharing on the screen so they can follow along with you or just to hear you read it directly to them (so they can clearly see your face). Take time throughout reading your letter to pause, check how your service user is engaging with the letter and whether or not they need you to stop if it feels too overwhelming. Upon completion of the letter, leave some time and space for reflection for the two of you. If the service user does not speak within this time, you may want to consider asking them how they found the letter, whether they had any particular thoughts or feelings in relation to it, and whether it was similar or different to what they expected. If you have a sense that there are similarities within the two of your letters, it is helpful to reflect on this, and consider how this exemplifies the joint journey the two of you have been on throughout therapy. For any variances within the letter, once again have time to think through why this may be the case and how you may have experienced things differently.

On the whole, the goodbye letters provide lasting transitional objects that the service user can take away with them to re-read outside of the sessions. Hamill et al. (2008) spoke of how service users continue to re-experience their letters as a direct message from their therapist about themselves. Prior to leaving the final session, it is helpful to check with the service user that they have copies of all the CAT tools that they require for their own personal use outside of the therapy.

Karen shares her own goodbye letter, which she shared with her therapist within the final session and then reflects on what it was like to say goodbye to the therapist as the session drew to an end.

Karen's Goodbye Letter to Therapist

Dear [Therapist],
As my therapy sessions come to an end, I would like to say how much I feel I have benefitted from it.

At first, I wasn't sure that I did really need therapy but soon realised that I was very anxious to bring situations to my sessions. However, now as the sessions are ending, I am aware that what I am bringing to the sessions I already have the answers to.

Therapy has given me a greater insight to really get to know myself. It has also helped me to understand other people more in a way that helps me to realise that my actions and the way I think and feel may not be how others act and feel.

I feel that I am now more patient and much more relaxed in myself. I tend to think things through now before I react. By doing this, my relationships with others are much improved.

The therapy at first did feel like a bit of an emotional roller-coaster as lots of things came up causing me to feel a little hurt and irate. However, I am pleased that I stuck with this as I have now come out the other side and can really see the benefits of the therapy.

I do feel you need to be at the right point in your life or illness to truly feel the benefit.

It's important to have a therapist you can easily work alongside, which is how I felt with yourself.

Thank you for giving me the opportunity of having therapy which I'm sure I will take with me for my future days and will find helpful for issues which may come along.
Thank you,
Karen

Karen says:

> *... that was my therapist's one concern, she knows that I do have attachment issues and she worried that we wouldn't be able to, you know, detach at the end of it. However it was absolutely fine I got her a card and a bottle of wine and I thanked her and we had a hug and we did end it and it did work but that was her one concern... because when she highlighted that, because I've got to prove to her that this isn't gonna happen and me getting stronger through therapy is gonna show that.*

Andrew reflects upon his goodbye letter, which he shared with the therapist and how after ten years since completing therapy, his feelings about the goodbye letter have changed.

Andrew says:

> *So, I don't recognise all the things I wrote in my letter, though now. I felt like*
> *I was blaming people for the way I am, and I don't necessarily think they*
> *were. I'm saying it's the way I'm wired and sort of looking back and quite a*
> *lot of things, you know, in, in sort of my life, it's like I'm spotting signs that*
> *I now know what to look for.*
>
> *I couldn't have got to this point without everything happening so I'm not*
> *gonna beat myself up that it's taken me 50 years to figure this out. It's just*
> *there's been a process and it's now I'm at the process where that bit's rele-*
> *vant and I can deal with it. I mean one of the big things I've done recently*
> *is that I've let go, I've let go of the past.*

What if the service user doesn't bring a goodbye letter?

Within the final session, if the service user expresses that they have been unable to write or bring a goodbye letter, it can be worth exploring with them the
reasons as to why this may be the case. There could be a number of reasons,
such as the service user has experienced a difficult week, is finding the ending
difficult, has completed an alternate way to mark the ending, finds writing
difficult, or is struggling to know what to write within the letter. Whatever the
case, having an open discussion about the reason for not writing the letter, in
a non judgemental, sensitive way, will help for further reflection surrounding
the ending. You may wish to ask the service user to imagine if they were to
have written a letter what it would have included. This will allow you to get
a sense of the service user's thoughts surrounding the journey of therapy,
what they have gained, how they feel about the ending, and how they will
manage outside of therapy. Once this discussion has been held, you can then
suggest the sharing of your own letter, followed by a shared discussion of
post-therapy growth.

What happens next?

Alongside the goodbye letters within the final session, you may also consider
with the service user the plan to meet again for the three-month review. We will
discuss the review itself in more detail in the next chapter. In planning this,
however, you may think in the final session with the service user about how
they will manage during the time between the end of the therapeutic contract
and the review session. To a certain extent, this may focus on relapse preven-
tion planning, reflecting together on how the service user will aim to keep an
observing eye on their problematic patterns; reminding themselves of their
exits which they have already found; and noting how they can continue to
revise problematic patterns over the course of the forthcoming weeks. In a way,
this is encouragement for the service user to practice being their own therapist.
Karen reflects here on the recognition that she was eventually able to do this:

Karen says:

> *Isn't it funny when you've had your therapy and you learn to make the con-*
> *nections yourself. Yeah, like you learn-Where did that ... you start asking*
> *yourself 'where that's come from?' – you do that to yourself.*

Outcome measures

An additional task that is often associated with the end of therapy is the repetition of any outcome measures that you may have invited the service user to
complete prior to the start of therapy. Some therapists may also complete these
measures midway through the block of therapy sessions, but for most, if they are
used, measures are completed at the beginning and end of therapy, and at the
follow up session. As outlined in Chapter 6, the main objective measures that are
used alongside a CAT therapy are the Inventory of Interpersonal Problems (IIP,
Horowitz et al., 1988) and the Personality Structure Questionnaire (PSQ,
Pollock et al., 2001). Depending on the setting or service you are working in,
you may of course also wish (or be required!) to use other generic symptom- or
wellbeing-based measures that aren't specific to CAT.

It can be difficult to know when precisely to ask the service user to repeat the
objective measures as you approach the end of therapy. If you chose to give
them to the service user to take away following the final session, there is the
question of how and when these will be returned to you and how best to feedback to the service user the results and an interpretation of them. It may be
easier to give them to the service user to take away following the penultimate
session, to be returned in the final session so that any changes between pre- and
post-therapy measures can be reflected on together. At times you may ask a
service user to complete them in the waiting room prior to coming into a session (if they are someone who tends to arrive early, and if the waiting room is
sufficiently quiet that they can do this without the possibility of someone looking over their shoulder!). You'll know the service user fairly well by this point
in therapy and will be able to negotiate with them what feels best.

If everything has gone well, you will both be hoping to see a reduction in the
scores on the outcome measures (indicating fewer interpersonal difficulties and
a greater degree of integration of elements of the self). Whilst both the IIP and
the PSQ will give you an overall score which you can compare with the pre-
therapy score to give a broad-stroke, quantitative indicator of change, it is
equally important to reflect with the service user on any changes within individual items and their subjective experience of this. This can really help to
illuminate where change has occurred and what might be left to work upon.

It's also not uncommon for scores on objective measures to have either (1)
not changed very much or (2) increased by the end of therapy, and it is of
course important to also think about what this may mean. Whilst this can feel
disheartening for both therapist and service user, there can be several reasons
for this. One of the things that we almost always remind service users of in our

goodbye letters is that it is not unusual to see symptoms returning to some degree around the end of therapy. As we've discussed above, the ending can provoke all sorts of feelings, including anxiety and anger, and whilst we hope that these can be named and worked through, it's not surprising that measures may reflect a sense of increased difficulty if the service user is in a more dysregulated state when completing them. It also may be, that other difficult life events have occurred separately around the ending of therapy that have cast the service user's sense of themselves in a more negative light. It is crucial to note that in some cases, as with any other intervention, therapy can be harmful – however, it would be important to name and address this as soon as it becomes apparent, so we would hope that scenarios where this comes to light only at the ending would be rare. Lastly, it is also surprisingly common that one of the stated aims of therapy (to increase recognition of and insight into problematic patterns and roles) results in higher scores on outcome measures completed towards the end of therapy because people have simply become more aware of their difficulties over time.

The evaluation of the outcome of therapy does, of course, not rest solely with the administration of objective measures. Whilst these can be incredibly useful tools to give an overall sense of change over time, the real outcomes are all of the changes you, the service user and their loved ones have noticed along the journey of therapy – changes that will no doubt continue to unfold for many years after the ending. These will be captured within the 'exits' on their map, within your goodbye letter(s) and in whatever other creative means or metaphors you chose to use. In terms of acknowledging improvement outside of outcome measures, Karen shares how her therapist highlighted her achievements with her.

Karen says:

> ...by the end of that therapy, when she [therapist] said 'go over now, you know, what you came to achieve' and she said, 'how do you feel now about the guilt you were carrying'? And I was like, 'what guilt?' and she said, 'you know about your mum' and I said, 'Did I really say that?' And she had to pull the notes out and so that proved just how much we work had done and how much I had worked on myself to totally get that feeling out of my mind.

Andrew shares how far he had come in therapy through noticing a change in his response to questions around suicidal ideation, which showed a huge improvement for him.

Andrew says:

> I mean even now I was quite proud of the last therapy session that I had where they ask do you have any thoughts of self-harm or suicide, it's the first time I've ever said 'no'. And I was really, really proud of myself that I did that. I don't spend every day now with kind of, you know, suicide's an option; it's not taking over my thoughts.

Conclusion

Endings can raise difficult feelings not only for the service user, but also for the therapist. Space within supervision to consider your goodbye letter and your own feelings in relation to the service user is necessary for you to process the ending. At times endings can also leave the therapist with challenging emotions, particularly if it resonates with one's own experiences. Having time to discuss these feelings within supervision will help you to manage them in a safe environment. An authentic response from the therapist within the goodbye session is always key, and therefore having time beforehand to reflect in supervision is essential.

The sharing of the goodbye letters within the final session can be a powerful experience for the service user, reiterating to them the journey they have come on and how far they have come within the sessions. Identifying areas of progress, challenge, and how the time following sessions may be experienced, is useful content for the goodbye letter.

References

Hamill, M., et al. (2008). Letters in Cognitive Analytic Therapy: The patients' experience. *Psychotherapy Research*, 18(5). https://doi.org/10.1080/10503300802074505

Horowitz, L. M., Rosenberg, S. E., Baer, B. A., Ureno, G., & Villasenor, V. S. (1988). Inventory of interpersonal problems: Psychometric properties and clinical applications. *Journal of Consulting and Clinical Psychology*, 56, 885–892. https://psycnet.apa.org/doi/10.1037/0022-006X.56.6.885

Jellema, A. (1999). Cognitive Analytic Therapy: Developing theory and practice via attachment theory. *Clinical Psychology and Psychotherapy*, 6(1), 16–28. https://doi.org/10.1002/(SICI)1099-0879(199902)6:1%3C16::AID-CPP182%3E3.0.CO;2-N

Mann, J. (1973). *Time-Limited Psychotherapy*. Harvard University Press.

Martin, E. S. & Schurtman, R. (1985). Termination anxiety as it affects the therapist. *Psychotherapy*, 22, 1. https://psycnet.apa.org/doi/10.1037/h0088532

Pollock, P. H., Broadbent, M., Clarke, S., Dorrian, A., & Ryle, A. (2001). Personality Structure Questionnaire (PSQ): A measure of the multiple self states model of identity disturbance in Cognitive Analytic Therapy. *Clinical Psychology & Psychotherapy*, 8(1), 59–72. https://doi.org/10.1002/cpp.250

Ryle, A. (1997). *Cognitive Analytic Therapy for Borderline Personality Disorder: The Model and The Method*. Wiley and Sons.

Ryle, A. & Kerr, I. (2002). *Introducing Cognitive Analytic Therapy: Principles and Practice of a Relational Approach in Mental Health*. Wiley and Sons.

Turpin, C., et al. (2011). What are the important ingredients of a CAT goodbye letter? *Reformulation*, Winter, 30–31.

14   Time for review

Introduction

Often within the final session of the CAT contract to therapy, a review meeting is planned. This chapter explores the process of reviewing how the service user is managing following the completed sessions. How to approach the review is considered, alongside the structure of the review sessions and how to know when to offer more. Finally, determining the service user's progress will be touched upon as a follow-up to the objective and subjective measures of well-being discussed in the previous chapter.

What is the intention of a review in CAT?

Early in the development of CAT, Ryle (1995) reported that post-therapy interviews should be in place to focus on reviewing Target Problem Procedures (TPPs), establish how accurately the map has been remembered, whether it has been used and whether revisions have been put into place. Time between the end of therapy and the review session in CAT offers the service user opportunity outside of the regular therapy structure to see how they cope and to continue to develop recognition and revision of their problematic patterns. The service user has space to practice being their own 'therapist', to use what they have learnt within therapy in their own time, outside of the therapy room.

The review appointment is further space to reflect after an intense piece of work (Turpin, 2019). Review sessions are not an extension of the therapy, nor are they a way of preventing the impact of the ending, through offering more sessions. They have a very specific purpose, aiming to consolidate the work and to check in on the service user's progress, post-therapy. Turpin (2019) speaks of the importance of the time following therapy to provide space to increase the service user's own confidence within themselves and to continue with the awareness and developments established through the therapy.

The review appointment should therefore offer space to the service user to reflect on life events occurring over the previous weeks, how they coped, whether or not they were able to manage difficult situations and whether they used CAT tools to aid their understanding of such situations.

DOI: 10.4324/9781003308256-14

What does the service user need?

In general, those who have had up to 16 sessions of CAT are offered one three-month follow up. Those who are offered 24 sessions of CAT are offered four follow-ups. These are usually offered at one, two, three and six months following the completion of therapy (Ryle, 1997). The four review sessions post-contract of 24 sessions were established following recognition of how difficult it can be to manage endings when there may be difficult feelings of abandonment or rejection. Whilst most CAT practitioners remain in line with this standard practice, no evidence is available to underpin the reasoning as to why these time frames are recommended.

It can be argued that having structure, through planning the review at the point of the final session, can promote containment and boundaries. With this in mind, it can therefore be reasoned that planning a review based on service user need, rather than these recommended time frames, is also important. There are no hard-and-fast rules as to what should be offered; therefore, gauging the service user's need within the final session can determine what reviews are required. It may be that the service user is ready for the ending, feels that time outside of therapy will be manageable, and thus a straightforward plan for a three-month follow-up can be agreed.

At times, the service user may raise challenges that will occur for them outside of the time frame of therapy, such as the anniversary of the death of a loved one. Thus, together it can be discussed if a sooner review is required, to check in and see how the service user has managed. On other occasions, at the point of review, it may be acknowledged that some further time is needed to consolidate recognition and revision, and thus a further review can be planned. There may be times in which you encounter the service user wanting more, when you as a therapist feel that the progress outside of sessions has been maintained. Ending following review can also be anxiety provoking for the service user, and thus it is important to discuss this openly and to recognise their ability to function with independence and autonomy outside of the therapy. Whatever the case, ensure that these discussions are held collaboratively with the service user and that decisions are made in their best interests. Karen shares the change in her perception of her difficulties and how she has learnt to manage this outside of sessions.

Karen says:

> *I think it just gets into your psyche what you learned and there's always bits of it just sat there. And even if a sudden thought comes to mind about the past, I think we can rationalise it more because there was a reason why and if you look at that, that's why it happened so make allowances and move on. That's what I tell myself to do, like accept what has happened.*
>
> *It's like when I wrote my book in 2017, would I have been able to do that before CAT because all those feelings that got evoked when writing my story start right from childhood to who I am now, I don't think I would have*

had the strength to do that, because that would have triggered a lot, but because I had dealt with all that in there, I was like, oh yeah I'm not bothered now, I'm not bothered who reads it and it really doesn't faze me at all.

Andrew reflects upon his review appointment, and how he shared with his therapist the ups and downs he had experienced outside of sessions.

Andrew says:

Even just going back two months afterwards knowing that you had that, but felt more able to handle it but as it was when we came back a couple of months later, I said well you know I'd like to tell you I've been fine the entire time but I actually haven't and she said I'm actually happier that you haven't and you've had a little wobble because then you can see how you deal with it. And that you wouldn't be a person if you didn't have that, so that's good.

How do I structure the review session?

As with the evidence on number of review sessions being limited, the 'how-to' of a review session is also largely absent within the literature. Recognising with the service user the remit of the review session is initially important (e.g., reminding them that the session is not an extension of the therapy, but more so to check in on their progress since the contract of therapy came to an end). In doing so, you can then agree on what to discuss within the follow-up session, through checking in with the service user: 'What would you like to get from the session today?'

As a CAT practitioner, you can feel reassured to enter the session with a flexible structure in mind, of areas you may wish to focus on, if the service user requires further direction. This can include:

- *How have things been for you since you finished your contract of CAT?*
- *Are there any areas where you have noticed you have improved, or found further exits to the CAT map?*
- *Have you found any times difficult? How did you cope with these? Can we identify these situations as problematic patterns on the CAT map?*
- *Have you actively used your tools (e.g., CAT map, letters, monitoring sheets), since you completed therapy?*
- *Have you noticed yourself developing into your own 'therapist'?*
- *Are there any other exits we need to add to the map?*
- *Is there anything we need to add to the healthy map?*
- *What happens now? What are the next steps for you? How do you feel about continuing to cope as you have done, outside of therapy?*

The review session is very much structured around the service user being able to openly reflect on their progress outside of therapy, alongside the challenges they have encountered. On the whole, it would not be expected that everything has been 'rosy' outside of therapy (unless the service user has a perfectionist trap, and you notice with them, that they are caught up within this, and feeling as though they have to tell you that everything has been great). A good rule of thumb for the CAT practitioner is to look out for both the areas of development and the areas of difficulty the service user has encountered and how they have overcome these. Prompts and reminders may be needed to use the tools and skills they have learnt in therapy, to help recognise the problematic patterns and to find useful exit strategies to these. You may wish to talk to the service user about finding an equilibrium, a place in which they can integrate the positives and the struggles within their day-to-day life, and find a healthy, 'good enough' position.

Closing the process of review

As the session draws to a close, you may have a sense of how the service user is feeling about their progress and the review. You too may have a sense of where the service user is at, in terms of their wellbeing, and whether any further follow-up is required or whether this will be the final planned session. If this is the final review, as you have already formally said 'goodbye' within the ending session, this is not the place to repeat this. Instead, it is best to summarise the service user's progress, acknowledge the normality of facing challenges and how far they have come across the previous months of work. As a result of this, you can therefore highlight that at this current point in time, no further reviews would be required, and consider this together with the service user, to determine their agreement with this. Alternatively, if you have already planned or feel that additional reviews would be beneficial, this can be agreed together.

Closing the review may not always be this straightforward. There can be times when further progress is limited, and there may be some disappointment that more could not be achieved. Discussions surrounding signposting to additional external support, if needed, can be helpful (e.g., charitable organisations). Alternately, consideration of the remit of this contract of therapy and requirement of more in the future, should the service user agree to it, can also occur. Therapy is generally not a one-off experience, and service users may engage in more in the future (whether from the same or a different psychological approach). It can be helpful to review the original aims and goals from the current contract to highlight what has been achieved. Whilst not all hopes and wishes can be fulfilled, there may be a time in the future when the service user wishes to engage in therapy with a different focus. In this instance, however, the service user needs time and space from the current contract of therapy, to process, internalise and continue to review their experience.

Conclusion

The review in CAT is not seen as an 'add-on' or an extra session, but time in which to truly reflect on the service user's progress outside of therapy. Having time away from the routine weekly appointments can give space for further development, recognition of problematic patterns and time to consider alternate exits. Given the limited literature in this area, CAT practitioners are guided to follow the original time frame for review, suggested by Ryle (1997), whilst holding in mind the person-centred nature of the approach and need to adapt and flex according to service-user need.

References

Ryle, A. (1995). *Cognitive Analytic Therapy: Developments in Theory and Practice.* Wiley.
Ryle, A. (1997). *Cognitive Analytic Therapy and Borderline Personality Disorder: The Model and the Method.* Wiley.
Turpin, C. (2019). Follow up in CAT. *Reformulation*, Summer, 28–28.

15 The challenges of Cognitive Analytic Therapy

Introduction

As we have moved through the differing stages you will encounter in the process of offering Cognitive Analytic Therapy (CAT) to a service user, we by no means consider this book to be a 'manual' of what to do and expect within CAT. As we hope you will have gathered by reading the book this far, our premise is to give you an understanding of how the different stages of CAT can be structured whilst strongly holding in mind the main underlying principles of working collaboratively with the service user, considering the therapeutic relationship at all times and working within a person-centred frame. Through taking this stance, we recognise that there can often be times as CAT practitioners in which we encounter challenges from within the therapeutic relationship itself. These challenges can feel unnerving, distressing and anxiety-provoking to a therapist and can take time and effort to find a suitable resolution. Within this chapter, we offer some of the common challenges that therapists face within CAT, the literature that underpins these occurrences, and how as CAT practitioners we may aim to manage them. Such challenges include when you feel you are missing a piece of the jigsaw, encountering a therapeutic rupture, managing times when a service user doesn't come and coping with difficult feelings triggered within yourself as a therapist.

When I'm missing a piece of the jigsaw

There can be times within the therapy when you realise that there may be important information about the service user's life that you are missing or haven't covered within the initial assessment. This can often occur whilst you are writing the reformulation letter, as you reflect upon the early life experiences in relation to the development of problematic patterns, and you realise that you have spoken little about a certain family member or time within the service user's life. This in itself may be just an oversight, but it is worth considering why you have missed this information in relation to the service user's narrative and problematic patterns. For example, do you notice that the service user has possible patterns of feeling detached or cut off? Or is there a

DOI: 10.4324/9781003308256-15

sense of disavowing feelings or splitting off from painful emotions? If so, it may be that the service user finds it difficult to articulate certain relationships and together there has been an unconscious avoidance of that particular aspect of their life.

If you do notice this as you are writing the reformulation letter, it may be worth tentatively naming the absence of information, for example:

> *As I am writing this letter, I notice that we haven't touched upon Dad, your rela-tionship with him, or what he was like as a person. This may be something we want to discuss in more detail together, to explore your feelings in relation to him and to think about where together we may have been on the map in overlook-ing this.*

In doing so, you are beginning to nudge the service user outside of their zone of proximal development (Vygotsky, 1978), to bring the conversation into the open and step out of the avoidance. Alternately, you may have already begun some early mapping together and developed a reciprocal role (such as dismissing-to-dismissed), and you may speak within the reformulation letter about being caught up within the role together, for example:

> *There may be times in which we too are caught within the map. I have noticed that we have spoken little about Dad within our time together so far, and it may be that we have been caught in the dismissing-to-dismissed role, putting off focussing on this relationship. This may be something we think about together within sessions to aim to step out of this role, allowing us to speak further about Dad.*

Whether naming the missing part of the jigsaw within the reformulation letter or verbally within the room, the aim is to strengthen the therapeutic rela-tionship over time and bring difficult conversations into the open so that the service user feels more able to share emotionally painful information.

Managing a therapeutic rupture

The concept of therapeutic ruptures, defined as a weakening or deterioration of the quality of the therapeutic alliance, is of course not unique to CAT. It would be inaccurate also to view the concept of ruptures through a wholly negative lens – as several authors have suggested (e.g., Horvath & Marx, 1990; Safran et al., 1990); ruptures are a normal part of the therapy process, and positive outcomes in therapy are often more closely associated with the suc-cessful management and repair of ruptures than with a smooth, linear progres-sion in the alliance. Safran et al. (1990, p.156) elaborate:

The successful resolution of an alliance rupture can be a powerful means of disconfirming the service user's dysfunctional interpersonal schema. While failure to adequately resolve an alliance rupture is likely to lead to poor outcome in psychotherapy, "The successful resolution of an alliance rupture can be one of the more potent means of inducing change".

In CAT terms, a rupture may come about when something the therapist has done (or is perceived to have done) aligns with a painful reciprocal role (RR) for the service user, if the therapist can recognise and explore this, there is a valuable opportunity for something different to follow. In order to resolve a rupture or a potential rupture, however, we first need to notice its occurrence. So, how do we know when a rupture is occurring? Safran et al., in their 1990 paper, outline key "*rupture markers*" (service user verbalisations or behaviours indicating the presence of distinctive underlying psychological processes). Amongst other things, these include verbal or non-verbal expressions of negative sentiments (for example, hostility or a verbal attack on the therapist's competence), over-compliance with the therapist (to mitigate against feared rejection) and "avoidance manoeuvres" (such as skipping from topic to topic, arriving late or cancelling sessions). They go on to propose some general principles for the resolution of ruptures, which shall be briefly reviewed here before we move on to consider in greater depth a CAT-specific model of rupture and repair.

Safran et al. (1990) situate the process of resolving ruptures within the context of what they refer to as "therapeutic metacommunication" (i.e., the process of talking about what is currently occurring within the therapeutic relationship). They outline the following principles as key in this process (the reader is directed to read the full paper for more detail – whilst some of the language we might use has moved on since the time the paper was written, it includes some incredibly helpful observations and insights on rupture resolution that have withstood the test of time):

1. Attending to ruptures in the alliance (by noting "*rupture markers*");
2. Awareness of one's own feelings as the therapist, which they argue are a useful "barometer" for the quality of the relationship and are crucial for step 3: if, for example, feelings of anger towards the service user are present but not identified, they may be communicated indirectly and unintentionally;
3. Accepting responsibility and acknowledging one's own role in the interaction as the therapist;
4. Empathising with the service user's experience – accurate empathy is likely to help the service user feel understood and therefore aid further exploration and support the service user in identifying feelings that they may not have been fully aware of;
5. Maintaining the stance of the "participant/observer" so that unhelpful patterns aren't repeated within the metacommunication.

Safran et al. (1990) went on to outline a preliminary model of the processes involved in rupture and repair, using Rice and Greenberg's (1984) task analysis method (this involved intensive observation of alliance ruptures in their sample). Bennett et al. (2006) also utilised the task analysis method in their detailed observations of threats to the therapeutic alliance in completed CAT therapy cases. Crucially, they highlight that in CAT, threats to the alliance are seen as problematic patterns within which the therapist is as active as the service user – in other words, the difficulty is not situated *within* the service user but seen as occurring in the relational space between the two. In examining enactments from CAT cases defined as having both good and poor outcomes, they proposed a process model of rupture resolution within CAT as follows:

1. Acknowledge – the therapist recognises that an in-session event has occurred and communicates this directly to the service user, e.g., How are you feeling about what is going on between us right now?
2. Explore – therapist and service user express and explore their perceptions and feelings surrounding the in-session event
3. Linking and explanation – here the therapist invites the service user to link feelings with their CAT formulation or proposes a link
4. Negotiation – understanding of the link is elaborated, the therapist explores doubts, invites disagreements and agrees to modifications
5. Consensus – agreement about the in-session event and its association to other relationships/origins in the past is reached
6. Understand and assimilate feelings that may have been warded off – helping the service user to experience these whilst explaining why they have been avoided
7. Further explanation – establishing the link between the identified relational pattern and the wider formulation
8. New ways of relating - in which alternatives to the identified pattern are explored (through, for example, discussion or role play)
9. Closure using the resolution of the enactment to illustrate that change is possible, whilst reaffirming the focus upon the therapeutic relationship.

The model does not suggest a sequential, linear movement through stages but recognises that cycling back and forth between stages may occur, and that the overarching principles of collaboration and non-collusion are threads that run throughout. Crucially, Bennett et al. (2006) discovered that "therapists in good outcome cases identified a very high proportion of alliance threatening enactments" and conclude that the successful resolution of these is dependent upon the therapist's ability to recognise them. The model is a useful framework to help therapists reflect on their processes within therapy sessions and to develop confidence and competence in responding to alliance ruptures.

We would emphasise the importance of attunement within the therapeutic relationship – being present and attentive to your own feelings and the communication of the service user will aid in the recognition of enactments (anecdotally, we both often experience this as a feeling in the body or a subtle shift in the feeling in the room). Being able to tentatively name and explore what seems to be occurring can feel anxiety provoking as we are often not used to engaging in this kind of metacommunication in other areas of life. However, as we have heard, the successful recognition and resolution of enactments can contribute greatly to a positive overall outcome in therapy.

What if the service user wants more?

We have touched (within Chapter 14) upon what happens if you come to the end of therapy and the service user is wanting more, particularly if they feel their progress outside of therapy has been limited. You may find, however, that at times you encounter a pull to offer more within the contract of therapy. This may be if the service user is finding therapy difficult, feeling extremely low in mood, or feeling anxious at having to 'go it alone' outside of therapy. This can often feel difficult as a therapist, as ultimately we are there to support the service user, provide care and have hope that things will improve for them. We can feel pulled into wanting to provide more and go along with the service user's requests in order to make them feel safe and cared for.

Inevitably, however, in doing so, we too may once again be being pulled onto the map. One of the greatest things we've learned as CAT practitioners is that when something feels difficult, slow down, try not to react and return to the map. The map is the tool that can lead to understanding and open conversations about what may be happening in the room. In this case, if the service user is wanting more, through returning to the map, you may be able to recognise with them the pull for others to rescue them when things feel tough or the fear of being alone and needing others to be close by their side. In being able to openly name problematic patterns that may aid understanding of this request from the service user, you will be able to identify how responding to the desire for more will ultimately lead to further fulfilment of the problematic pattern. Your goal together is to step out of these patterns and to come to an agreement as to why offering more is not so beneficial.

Through such discussions you are aiming to maintain the boundaries of the contract of therapy. This in itself creates a safe and secure base for the service user to know what is offered will be maintained, and that through agreeing to more, you would be maintaining a problematic pattern, and in the long run reinforcing the belief in the service user that they wouldn't have managed without this having been offered. This could then be added to the map as an exit itself.

What if the service user doesn't come?

There may be times that the service user fails to attend an appointment, without cancelling or informing you of their whereabouts. This can be difficult with service pressures and policies which suggest one or two 'did not attends' (DNAs) must lead to discharge from the service. In therapy itself, this at times can feel rejecting of the service user, if this were to be followed without taking time to think psychologically, using the CAT map, to understand why the service user may be finding it difficult to attend.

As mentioned above, non-attendance to a session may be considered as a therapeutic rupture in itself. The missed sessions may come after a break in therapy (for example if the therapist has been on annual leave, or off work sick), whether planned or unforeseen. It may be that the break leads to feelings of separation anxiety as discussed in Chapter 13 (see Glenn, 1971, for further reflection on separation anxiety), where the service user experiences the gap in sessions as rejecting, and thus in turn rejects the following sessions.

Alternately, there may have been a hard conversation or occurrence in the previous session, which makes it hard for the service user to attend, and thus leads to them missing the session. Whatever the case, it is important for the therapist to take a step back and consider the service user's CAT map and what might be happening relationally between the two.

Reaching out to the service user through a letter to try to encourage them back to therapy is a useful technique to aim to step out of the RRs and to find a way to re-engage the service user within the sessions. Using a non-critical, non-threatening approach to such a letter is important in these cases, alongside a potential hypothesis of what may be happening within the therapeutic relationship. An example of this is as follows:

> I was sorry not to see you in our planned session today. I do wonder if it has felt difficult to return today following my unexpected sickness absence and having to cancel our previous session together. I wonder if in some way I left you feeling rejected, through having to cancel and not having our routine time in therapy? If this is the case, I hope that we can come back together to discuss your feelings in more detail, and to work through this jointly to find a good enough resolution for us to continue sessions.

It is hoped that in receiving such a letter, the service user feels able to come back to the next session, safe enough to explore their feelings in the context of a collaborative discussion and to reflect on what has happened in relation to the CAT map.

What if the service user's experiences trigger painful feelings for me?

As anyone who has been working as a psychological therapist for any length of time will no doubt tell you, experiencing painful feelings in relation to the work we do is – at some point – inevitable. There are several different levels at which this may occur of course. As therapists, we are privileged to bear witness to and share in incredibly powerful and moving moments with our service users. However, we are, by definition of the role, also likely to hear about and witness the consequences of some of the very worst things that human beings do to each other. Aside from any particular resonance with our own life experiences, this alone is likely to trigger painful feelings for us at times – and we would encourage you to notice and recognise this in yourself as well as use this as a source of empathy for the service user. This is of course an entirely natural and understandable response and something it will be important to name and seek support for within your own clinical supervision. Sometimes, when it may benefit them or the work, it can also be appropriate to share your feeling responses with the service user – again, this is something best discussed in supervision to explore (1) your own motivations for doing so and (2) how this may be experienced by the service user, given what you know of them and their map so far.

If we think of this as the first level of emotional response, the second level involves times when you share a key relational experience, presenting difficulty or traumatic event with your service user. Of course, you may not always be aware of this before the work begins, or even until you are a little way into the work, and that is perhaps a situation which requires a different level of consideration (see level 3, below). However, what if you are aware *before* picking up a case that one of these resonances applies and you anticipate that it will trigger painful feelings for you? Should this be a case that you perhaps ask a colleague to work with instead of seeing this service user yourself? Unsurprisingly, there are no "hard and fast" rules about this. Your decision is likely to be informed by (1) your sense of how far you have been able to process your own experiences in this regard, (2) how 'live' your own experiences are at the present time and (3) the level of safe, containing supervisory support you currently have available to you.

It probably goes without saying that there are times when we might need to take time off, step away from direct therapeutic work and seek help for ourselves. If this isn't the case, though, you might want to reflect on the pros and cons or the risks and benefits of taking on a case that has a significant resonance with your own story. It's worth remembering that even if you have experienced something very similar, the service user may have an entirely different experience of, response to and meaning attached to their experience than you have to yours. Having lived experience of trauma, discrimination, problematic relational patterns or our own physical or mental health difficulties as a therapist *does not* make us any less of a therapist; in fact, we would argue that your lived experience can be a strength – whilst no two experiences are the same, the level of compassion, empathy and understanding you can bring will be unique. Having said that, if you feel that working with *this person at this time* might be detrimental for your own wellbeing or might result in a less-containing therapeutic experience for them, it might be best to ask a colleague to work with them instead.

The third level to consider is the scenario whereby you are already working with someone when it becomes apparent that either (1) you have in common very similar presenting difficulties or traumatic life experiences or (2) their map and reciprocal role patterns are unhelpfully and powerfully connecting with your own. With regards to the latter point – do bear in mind that when recipro-cal roles or problem procedures are strong (even if they are in no way similar to your own), you are likely to be pulled "onto the map" at some point – this is a normal part of the therapeutic process and, as we have outlined already, is often a very useful experience to reflect upon, once you have disentangled your-self from it. We are referring here to those times when there is a 'meshing' of patterns or roles, so that you find yourself, again and again, in the bottom end of a role that is a very painful place for you or being pulled to react in a way that is all too familiar but ultimately unhelpful. We cannot emphasise enough the importance of the use of good clinical supervision in these cases. Whether that is because you have uncovered an experience of the service user's that pain-fully resonates with your own or whether your maps are 'entangled', you will need containing and consistent support from a supervisor who is experienced in relational working and with whom you have a safe enough relationship. As part of CAT practitioner training, all aspiring therapists are required to engage with their own CAT therapy (it's worth noting this isn't the case for all therapy trainings), and this experience can be invaluable in working through your own painful life experiences and developing a good enough sense of your own pat-terns and roles, so that you have a fighting chance of stepping back from them when they are triggered in a therapeutic context. As a therapist working in a relational model, you are in effect using yourself as a tool in doing the work of therapy, so it makes sense to keep this tool as well maintained as possible!

Conclusion

Difficult situations in therapy are inevitable. For any of us within a relationship with another, things do not always run 100 per cent smoothly. We can always face hiccups, arguments or disagreements within our relationships. With regards to resolution of the difficult situation, we can either fall into the trap (where we may gain temporary relief, but the pattern predictably happens again in the future) or we can seek an exit, through stepping back and considering what has happened, what was likely to happen if you followed the same behav-iour as usual and how to do something different. This chapter considers some of the challenges we at times face within the therapeutic relationship and endeavours to aid practitioners in seeking resolution. This list of challenges is by no means exhaustive and there may be many a time in which you face a concern, difficulty or obstacles within your relationships. The key message from us is to take your time, return to the map and endeavour to work collab-oratively to gain understanding of the rupture.

References

Bennett, D., Parry, G., & Ryle, A. (2006) Resolving threats to the therapeutic alliance in Cognitive Analytic Therapy of borderline personality disorder: A task analysis. *Psychology and Psychotherapy: Theory, Research and Practice*, 79(3), 395–418. https://doi.org/10.1348/147608305X58355

Glenn, M. L. (1971). Interpretation: Theory and practice. *Family Process*, 10(1), 123–132.

Horvath, A. O. & Marx, R. W. (1990). The development and decay of the working alliance during time-limited counselling. *Canadian Journal of Counselling*, 24(4), 240–260.

Rice, L. N. & Greenberg, L. S. (1984). Future research directions. In L. N. Rice & L. S. Greenberg (Eds.), *Patterns of Change: Intensive Analysis of Psychotherapy Process*. 289–308. Guilford.

Safran, J. D., Crocker, P., McMain, S., & Murray, P. (1990). Therapeutic alliance rupture as a therapy event for empirical investigation. *Psychotherapy: Theory, Research, Practice, Training*, 27(2), 154–165. https://doi.org/10.1037/0033-3204.27.2.154

Vygotsky, L. S. (1978). *Mind in Society: The Development of Higher Psychological Processes*. Harvard University Press.

16 Author and service user reflections

Introduction

In true CAT style, we wanted to provide an ending to the book that incorporates a narrative of reflection, experience and emotion. Karen and Andrew have written their own reflections on the process of being involved in the book, what this (and CAT) has meant to them and what benefit they hope it will have to you as the reader. We (Sarah and Jayne) wanted to give a little insight into what the experience of writing the book has been like for us, and how we hope it goes some way in bridging a gap which we felt was apparent during our own training in the model.

Service user reflections

Karen's final words

As I reflect on my involvement with this book, I feel really privileged to have been invited to have my input. I feel it is so important for the beginning therapists reading this to see the true impact that CAT can have on a person's life. I hope it has allowed them to see that it isn't plain sailing, and it asks an awful lot from the individual. In doing so, I hope that it shows the support and dedication needed from the therapist to keep their service user on track and be with them every step of the way, especially for the times when the going really does get tough. However, I'm sure they will realise that with patience and dedication, this therapy can make a huge difference in a very beneficial way.

I certainly feel it has done this for me. I often reflect on my therapy and constantly remind myself that I am 'good enough'. I also tell myself that if others are not happy with me or the decisions that I make, then that also is fine, as I must remember that I am not going to be 'liked' by everyone. What is most important to me is that I remain well and if this means being assertive in saying no to things that are going to have an impact on me then that is what I must do. In realising this though, through my therapy, I have taught myself to show my assertiveness in a calm and controlled manner. My therapy helped me to find it within myself to do this and I feel much happier for managing to accomplish this.

DOI: 10.4324/9781003308256-16

My life is now much calmer. Although my therapy was quite some time ago now, it shows how it was so valuable to me.

As I continue my life journey, at times when I may feel overwhelmed, I always take a pause and reflect on just what I learned in that period. I requested therapy for several reasons, and I'm pleased that it certainly had the outcome that I hoped for. However, therapy is not something you can do and then just forget about it and then expect your life to change for the better; it is something that requires you to constantly put the work in. You are the only one who can change how you live your life; your therapist can just provide you with the tools to assist you to make those changes.

I sincerely hope that CAT is offered to lots more people as when I often listen to older people who are struggling in coming to terms with who they are, to have this would certainly shed some light on why they are who they are and perhaps why they have learned certain behaviours. To go back to their younger selves and the life they have lived can only help them to make changes they need to in order to enjoy a more fulfilled and happy life. Therefore, I hope that all this is taken into consideration when referrals are made for CAT as to go into such depth of your life can truly make a huge difference going forward.

It is important that people know what CAT is; therefore, the word needs to get out to the public as very few people seem to even know this exists. They cannot request something that they have never heard of, so perhaps it is time that the health professionals thought of ways that this can be promoted. To have successful therapy leading to a much happier life can surely only be of benefit to our NHS in the future.

I've thoroughly enjoyed working alongside the authors in the publishing of this book. I feel it will be a huge benefit to the reader. It explains the concept of CAT with such clarity. It is so refreshing that the book shares personal stories both from the authors and those with lived experience. It explains every detail of the process of CAT, and I believe that even those who are looking into CAT for the very first time will have no problems in following this and understanding every step of the process.

The fact that the book has been written by those who thoroughly understand CAT both from a clinical point of view and those on the receiving end of the therapy can only reassure beginning therapists that they are learning from the very best. This will hopefully enrich their journey!

Andrew's final words

Talking about my CAT and reading through this book has been an interesting time. It would be fair to say that it saved my life. Not in a dramatic way; it has given me the tools to help me live my life. I would like to say I lived happily ever after, but real life isn't like that. I have realised during this experience how much of CAT is still part of my everyday life, how I use it to navigate life's problems and challenges. I actually hear the sat-nav voice in my head at times.

I have had many therapies since my CAT, but it was experiencing it which has made the other therapy work. Things click into place now.

CAT is a powerful therapy that in my opinion is underused. That said, it is definitely not a first step for anyone. I believe I needed to be 'in the right place' in order for it to work. CAT is hard work; even from the first week I was never sure whether I would return for the next week's session.

I had forgotten a lot of what was involved in some of the therapy. I guess we all take what we find most useful and discard that which we don't.

Where am I now then?

I was diagnosed a few years ago with Fibromyalgia, which has been a rather large spanner in the works, not least with my depression and anxiety. I have had to get used to my new normal, my limitations and living with chronic pain. I will always need therapy to cope with this but that's fine, I'm happy with that. I take medication and will be on it for life, so the occasional therapy is no big deal. I realise that it all seems a bit doom and gloom. It isn't; it just has challenges.

In the plus column of life, I have rather a few ticks. I paint and have been lucky enough to sell some; mostly, though I give my paintings away, mostly because it makes me feel good.

I have been involved with various Fibromyalgia groups. One such group is Rock Off Fibro, we have released to date a double CD featuring 36 tracks from various bands including a song I wrote and sang backing vocals on; oh, and I did the artwork for the front cover of the album. We have also released a DVD which features videos of the artists, some of which were recorded at our Rock Off Fibro concerts, I am the 'cover star' on that DVD. We have had an art exhibition and will hopefully be having another concert in the near future. I have had my artwork featured on several musicians' releases which has been a dream come true. I have recorded and released an experimental album, a real DIY affair but I have enjoyed every minute.

I have been involved with Teesside University on their doctorate program as a service user representative. I have helped with research, been part of the interview panel and shared my experiences with the trainees.

I think though my biggest success to date is what is to come. I have enrolled on an Access to Higher Education course at my local college, the ultimate aim is to go to university and get a degree in Psychology.

Something that has occurred to me recently is how I gauge what is success. In the past it would mean I was good at my job; now it's more about how I feel. Am I happy? Yes. Success. It's as simple as that. I am married to my soul mate and best friend; I have two grown-up children who I have a great relationship with. I am winning at life. That is a small sentence, but I need to repeat it, in italics: *I am winning at life*. If that doesn't tell you about my state of mind, then nothing will.

I have felt honoured to have been a small part of this book, definitely another tick in the winning-at-life column. It has been a pleasure to be involved. I hope you, the reader, get as much from it as I have.

Author reflections

Sarah's final words

As we have come to the 'last' chapter of the book, I've been reflecting frequently about the forthcoming ending. In true CAT practitioner style, coming to an end is something I often give much thought to, particularly when there has been great investment in what I am saying goodbye to. My mind has been circling with thoughts of 'what will it be like to no longer be writing the book each week?' 'I'll miss my writing sessions with Jayne'. 'We have been so fortunate to have two truly amazing people involved in sharing their lived experience within the book; how can we thank them enough?' 'How can we mark the ending?'.

No doubt, from my thoughts, you can then picture the flurry of emotions I've been having, to moments of great joy and achievement seeing the book form to feelings of sadness as I lose the more frequent connection with the people invested with me in making this book a success. I was reflecting more recently that often people use the term 'blood, sweat and tears' to depict the intense work and effort that goes into ventures such as this. However, for me that doesn't ring true. I have been afforded the opportunity to write this book with my best friend. Jayne and I met through work, as assistant psychologists, some 20 years ago and have been close friends ever since. Our professional lives have frequently crossed paths, through completing our doctoral training together, working in separate specialties but then going on to complete our CAT training together, Jayne coming to work for a year on secondment within the Older Adults directorate where I was working, having the same CAT supervision group for a number of years, and more recently working together once again on the Doctorate in Clinical Psychology course at Teesside.

The solidity of our relationship (and also the yin and yang of our personalities) has meant that the process of writing this book (for me at least!) has been a truly rewarding one. We have been able to debate concepts and opinions together, respect each other's differing views and working styles and appreciate each other's desire to want to write different sections in the book. Although it's been a challenge, finding time in busy schedules to write, managing both work and family life, as well as our own personal ill health at times, it hasn't felt like 'blood, sweat and tears'. It has been an enjoyable challenge, one which we are jointly passionate about and hope that it will help many of you training in CAT. It is something we had always felt was missing in the literature, and it has been a huge feat for both of us to be able to say that it is something we have produced.

Karen and Andrew have also been central to making this book so enjoyable to write. They came into our lives through their work as Service User and Carer Representatives at Teesside University. We worked with them for a number of months before we ever came to know they had previously had CAT and what they thought about it. When they did share their experience of CAT, we knew we had to approach them to see if they wanted to be involved in the book. We have had some great times together during the process (the day spent interviewing them both at a lovely hotel being one) and difficult times too (as we sat together and shared lived experiences and felt the emotional sadness for one another). Without Karen and Andrew, however, this book wouldn't be as accessible, engaging and as true to life as it is. We are truly thankful to you both, and as I've said in many an email before, you are both absolute *stars*!

I fly the flag for CAT in all of the work that I do, and I hope that this enthusiasm comes through in the book. CAT has multiple levels of utility. Relationships are central to all that we do and in every aspect of our lives! I hope that your relationship with this book helps in developing skills in what I feel is a really engaging, dynamic and effective approach!

Jayne's final words

As I reflect back on the process of writing this book, I am reminded of the feelings of initial excitement we experienced on learning that our 'pitch' had been successful – this was closely followed by the recognition of the enormity of what we had taken on and a sincere wish to do this work justice. In essence, we hoped to write the book that we ourselves wished we, as beginning CAT practitioners, had had.

Our writing 'process' often began with dialogue – conversations, debates and reflections upon our experience of CAT both as therapists and as service users – before we settled on the overall structure for each section and made a plan for the content. It was a pleasant surprise to realise that we were drawn to writing different aspects of each chapter and that where we had differing views, we were always able to find a way forward.

I feel immensely grateful and lucky to have been able to co-create this text with Karen, Andrew and Sarah. Without Sarah's drive and dedication, this work simply would not have happened. Karen and Andrew have been courageous and authentic in sharing their own stories and experiences of CAT and I hope that you as the reader are as moved by their accounts as we were in reading and hearing them.

As you will have gathered by now, the idea of the relationship is central to our understanding of CAT, and this has also been true of my experience of authoring this book with Sarah. When, towards the end of our writing process, I found myself back on my own map, Sarah's voice was the one that helped me to find my way back onto steadier ground. The work we do as therapists is hard, and above all else I implore you to stay connected to the relationships, both within and outside of work, that help to nurture you and keep you steady, both during the fair weather and during the stormy times in life. My hope is that this book will provide you with a rudder (or, in Andrew's words, a sat-nav!) to help steer and guide your beginning journey with CAT. Ultimately, I hope that working within this profoundly relational model brings you a wealth of connected moments throughout your career.

Summary

As we come to a close, we want to remind you of what we feel is the central part to CAT – the relationship. Being a therapist can be challenging, and you can often be left holding uncomfortable emotions. Always take time to step back, reflect, return to the map and make sense of what may be going on for you and the service user. Use regular supervision to think through your work, be open to exploration and immerse yourself in the evidence base and literature surrounding CAT. We wish you well in your journey of training!

Index

Pages in *italics* refer to figures.